BODY and ANTIBODY

BODY *and*
ANTIBODY

A REPORT ON THE
NEW IMMUNOLOGY

David Wilson

Alfred A. Knopf   New York   1972

THIS IS A BORZOI BOOK
PUBLISHED BY ALFRED A. KNOPF, INC.

FIRST EDITION

to Elizabeth

Contents

Preface

With the benefit of hindsight, I now realise that the genesis of this book occurred in the City of Exeter in September 1969. In the course of earning my living as a television and radio science reporter for the BBC News, I was covering the annual meeting of the British Association for the Advancement of Science. This strange function originated in the first half of the nineteenth century, when people like T. H. Huxley were pioneering not only the social usefulness of "science," but also the scientific view of ourselves and our existence based on Darwin's newly propounded views on the origin of all species including mankind. These men decided that "science" needed a shop window and they founded the British Association and its annual meeting. At this meeting, scientists were to present their latest results to a general audience of other scientists and interested laymen; here matters of scientific moment could be discussed among intelligent, but not necessarily specialist, groups; here, converts to science could be made. This example was followed in the United States too, where the American Association for the Advancement of Science likewise holds an annual public meeting, going on for a week at least.

Perhaps the original enthusiasts had not digested Darwin's theories well enough, for what has happened since is that "science" has evolved rapidly and split up into innumerable highly specialised branches; while their annual meetings have developed but slowly into gigantic, lumbering, ill-controlled monsters. The practising scientist nowadays announces his new results and his important discoveries at specialist meetings and symposia of his own discipline. It is at these meetings and in the specialist scientific journals that new theories are battled over. But the two Associations for the Advancement of Science continue to present enormous packages of simultaneous lectures and discussions covering every type of scientific work, as well as the impacts of science on society. It all becomes most confusing. Even the most experienced journalist finds it quite impossible to know whether there will be the better story in "Engineering" or "Education"; or how to choose between "Zoology," "Psychology," and "Mathematics."

Towards the end of that sunny week in September among the new buildings of the rapidly expanding University of Exeter, suffering from mental indigestion and that weariness of the legs caused by toiling up and down the steep though rounded hills of Devonshire, I was irritated when the producer of one of the programs for which I work asked me to provide a brief summing-up. I protested, not for the first time, that this was impossible from the very nature of the meeting. This particular producer, being a very reasonable man, saw my point of view and changed his request. He asked instead for a short piece on the subject I thought had emerged as the most interesting on the present "frontiers of knowledge." Furthermore, he was prepared to give me the rarest gift of all in my job—time to think before preparing my broadcast.

I concluded that immunology was the most exciting of the scientific disciplines at the moment, by which I mean it was the one that excited me the most by the fresh insights it is providing into so many of the current problems.

If I were to list the names of all who have helped me since then and provided information for this book, it would sound suspiciously like name-dropping. It might also appear to be a journalistic trick to bolster with such eminent names and grave authorities the inadequacies of a mere reporter's view of a great scientific discipline.

I hope therefore that it will be enough to state that no man or woman who works in the field of immunology has refused to see me when I have approached them or denied me any piece of information or any minute of time that I have requested. The list of those who have given me particularly great help is therefore the list of those I have pestered the most. First I must thank Dr. James Mowbray, reader in immunopathology at St. Mary's Hospital Medical School in London, because he was the first person I went to for help and because he has given me detailed assistance by reading and amending the most technical parts of this book. Then I must mention Dr. John D. Humphrey, deputy director of the National Institute for Medical Research at Mill Hill, and his colleague Dr. Avrion Mitchison. Dr. David Owen, secretary of the Medical Research Council, provided me with particularly valuable guidance when I was most a stranger to the new country. Professor J. R. Batchelor, of Queen Victoria Hospital, East Grinstead, not only provided his quota of information and help but was also responsible, although he doesn't know it, for interesting me in the subject in the first place. Sir Peter Medawar is another scientist who does not realise how much he is responsible for this book, but it was he who fired me with my first interest in his subject, and it was also he who made me a convert to Sir Karl Popper's philosophy of science. There is no doubt that in the U.S.A. the people I must thank are Professor Robert Good and his wife, Dr. Joanne Finstad (who is also his scientific colleague). They provided me, though a complete stranger, with every scrap of information I could want at the first request.

For technical background and factual reference, I have

mainly relied on *Immunology for Medical Students,* by Humphrey and White (third edition, London: Blackwell; 1969), and *An ABC of Modern Immunology,* by E. J. Holborow, much of which originally appeared as a series of articles in *The Lancet,* and which was published in booklet form by *The Lancet* Limited (London, 1968). Thanks for permission to print quotations to the publishers of *Changing Patterns,* by Sir Macfarlane Burnet (London: Heinemann; 1968); *Conjectures and Refutations,* by Karl Popper (London: Routledge; 1963); *Induction and Intuition in Scientific Thought,* by Sir P. Medawar (London: Methuen; 1969); *Margin of Safety,* by John Rowan Wilson (London: Collins; 1965); article on Immunology by Dr. J. D. Humphrey, (*HMSO, Annual Report of the Medical Research Council 1968/69*).

It is customary to exonerate all those who have provided assistance from any blame for the author's errors. I heartily endorse the custom, but I cannot honestly add the other usual remark, "Thanks to my wife, without whose patience . . ." etc. If my wife had not suddenly involved herself in the teaching of Tudor and Stuart history and continually interrupted my writing to discuss the religious settlement of Queen Elizabeth and the failure of Cromwell's Parliaments, this book would have been finished much sooner.

—DAVID WILSON

Hampton Hill
December 1970

BODY *and* ANTIBODY

Chapter 1

Defining the
Science of Self

One of the most profound insights into our own bodies, na-
tures, and relationships with all living things in our world
yielded by science is the theory that there is a physical basis
of individuality. This means that there are some molecules,
some combinations of atoms, which are mine, and mine
alone, possessed by no other human being or animal. Furthermore, these "personal" molecules are no individual quirk.
My body uses the unique pattern provided by them to define
myself, to acknowledge what is part of "me," and to recognise the essential threat in all that is not "me."

The origins and invention of this theory, its development,
the production of evidence to support it, its use to explain
the workings of the body, its practical application in clinical
medicine, the new approach it has provided in the assault on
yet-unconquered diseases and problems—all this I have
called the "science of self." Among scientists the discipline is
known as immunology, but this is as inadequate as a human
surname is in describing the person who bears it. The word
"immunology" and the human surname tell us only something about the forebears from which they came.

This science of self is a creation of the last twenty years, and has been overshadowed all its life by the more glamorous, more far-ranging, but less practically productive science of molecular biology. The two disciplines are closely interrelated. In many ways they are contemporaries and have cross-fertilised each other, but naturally molecular biology has provided a foundation, both imaginative and experimental, for the more particularised immunology. Molecular biology has provided the greatest intellectual and imaginative development of our time: an explanation in physical and chemical terms for the extraordinary variety of life forms we observe on our planet, and a vision of the mechanism by which like breeds like.

"Man and lions, eagles and pheasants, the horned deer . . ." wrote Chekhov, and went on down the scale of life as far as the starfish. We know now that he should have gone much farther and included invisible bacteria, plankton, algae, and viruses if he wished to indicate all the forms that life can take. Molecular biology has identified the organisational mechanism that is common to all life forms—the nucleic acids.

The central thesis of molecular biology is that all life on our planet is the organisation of atoms and molecules performed by the nucleic acids DNA and RNA. These "acids" (another uninformative word) are in fact molecules, consisting of enormously long chains of atoms, essentially spiral, or helical, in shape. At regular intervals along the entire length of this spiral structure are subunits, just four different types for each of the two nucleic acids. The order in which these subunits are placed, from one end to the other of the spiral backbone, both produces and defines the life form that we see. In other words, the difference between a human being and a rhubarb plant is the difference in the order in which four different groups of atoms are arranged on some very long spiral molecules. Essentially, the nucleic acid that defines and produces a zebra, say, is capable of organising around itself, a reproduction of itself—which therefore defines and produces another zebra.

We have as yet no convincing, conclusive explanation of how the first nucleic acids were formed or found on the planet earth. But the beginning of life was the first self-reproduction by one of them.

From a scientific point of view, it is therefore reasonable to see all the teeming life on the surface of our planet as a competition between these spiral molecules. They compete for the control of the chemical substances available in that thin shell that we see as the interface between rock, water, and atmosphere, but that could also be described as the approximately spherical shell where the density of atoms on a globular collection of matter suddenly decreases rapidly.

We do not know whether life began with the simplest and shortest of the spiral molecules. These comparatively simple, short stretches of nucleic acid organise only very simple collections of chemicals around themselves. We know them as viruses. Since they cannot reproduce themselves without the aid of the structures formed by longer and more complex nucleic acids, it is quite possible that they are degenerate forms developed later in the history of evolution. Yet they have undoubted efficiency in "pirating" the chemicals organised by longer types of spiral nucleic acid: they then use these chemicals to reproduce themselves, as we have all experienced when suffering from a virus disease.

The most important stage in the development of the spiral molecules on earth was when they organised the chemicals around themselves so as to form a continuous protective covering. Each spiral molecule produces a membrane that can contain supplies of the chemicals it needs and within which it can develop structures to maintain the whole, repair the various parts, and build up the materials needed for the reproduction of the central spiral molecule itself. This organisation we call the cell.

Molecular biology then sees the development of even longer chains of nucleic acid, with greater numbers of the four subunits able to provide further instructions for organisation. Thus the reproduction of the spiral molecule inside its cell membrane leads to the formation of other cells, each containing an identical spiral molecule at its center, forming a fresh nucleus. From this develop groups of cells, each cell having inside it an identical spiral molecule. The groups cooperate to form a multicellular organism, taking in even more of the surrounding chemicals and using them to sustain, preserve, and increase the number of spiral molecules, all exactly the same as the one that started the group.

After this comes a group in which different cells perform different functions. Each cell contains, again, an identical copy of the original spiral molecule. But by now it is so long and carries so many subunits that it is capable of making different cells perform different functions by using only part of its organisational powers in each cell. Certain lengths of arranged subunits are either switched off or blocked off so that the instructions they carry for the operation of a liver cell are not used if that particular cell happens to be, say, a kidney cell.

By the time we reach the higher animals there are many spiral molecules within the nucleus of each cell. We can regard these as one immensely long spiral molecule broken up into shorter lengths for convenience, or just, possibly, as groupings of spiral molecules that have somehow "learned" to cooperate. But the essential thing is that in every one of our cells there is an identical collection of these spiral molecules, with a total of millions upon millions of arranged subunits along their spiral spines. Every cell contains all the instructions necessary to organise the formation and working of every other cell. In the course of this organisation of the collection of thousands of millions of cells that become a human being, the process of cell differentiation has been initiated. It continues under instruction from the nucleic acids, so that the liver cells, using only part of the information carried by these acids, are already behaving as liver cells, rather than brain or nerve or kidney cells. It still seems, however, that the objective is to organise as many of the immediately surrounding chemicals as possible in order to preserve and maintain the nucleic acid in the cells and to reproduce it.

Think how we take in the chemicals of the atmosphere when we breathe, and how we fight anything that tries to stop this. Each of us seizes upon the chemicals already organized and collected from both the atmosphere and the ground by the nucleic acid of, for example, the cabbage, and converts them to our own nucleic acid preservation.

Human beings certainly seem to be the latest, and perhaps the final, organisation produced by the spiral molecules. We named the nucleic acids thousands of years after we had named ourselves, millions of years after the first of our type of nucleic acid had appeared. And we have coined the names "zebra" and "lion," "eagle," "pheasant" and "horned deer" for the organisations produced by groups of spiral molecules in which the order of the subunits differs from our own and differs again among themselves.

The concept of "fitness" in the evolutionary sense is familiar to all of us. The great attraction of the central thesis of molecular biology is that it not only provides a chemical or physical conception of the basic facts of life, such as like breeding like, but also fits in so neatly with our already developed concepts of the evolution and development of our world. Fitness then becomes a measure of the differing abilities of nucleic acids to organise the chemicals around them for their own survival and reproduction in competition with other nucleic acids. More correctly, fitness is a measure of the competitive ability of one ordering of subunits along a nucleic acid against another ordering. The competition is not always a direct striving of one against another for the same chemical molecule. We consume plant excretions in the shape of oxygen; plants consume our excretions in the shape of carbon dioxide.

Competition between species—the lion eating the zebra —is easily seen in terms of competition between different spiral molecules. Yet long stretches of lion nucleic acid will appear very similar to stretches of zebra nucleic acid in the arrangement of the subunits. Many of the body chemicals of a lion are very like those of a zebra. Lion flesh, blood, and liver closely resemble those of a zebra; consequently, those lengths of subunits which order these organizations in the two animals will be very similar. Cannibalism and warfare among men can be looked at from the same point of view. Here the nucleic acids of the two competitors are even more alike; the differences in the ordering of the subunits will only be such as to define the distinctions between two warring tribes or even between two different families. Putting it the other way about, the absolute similarity between two stretches of subunits gives my children certain features which they have recognisably inherited from me; where they differ from me is where the order of subunits on my wife's nucleic acid has prevailed.

But this kind of competition between super-aggregations of cells organised into rival animals is comparatively crude. Both lions and ourselves face competition for vital chemicals from single-celled organisms like bacteria and from the viruses, which do not even have a cell wall. These things we cannot club, shoot, or tear apart.

Our nucleic acids have had to develop a means of defense against the pirate activities of other types of nucleic acid in

the course of evolution, just as they have had to develop the
whole organism into something capable of resisting the attacks of other whole organisms. If they had not developed
both these forms of resistance, they would not have been fit
in the evolutionary sense and we would not exist. It would
appear simple for a nucleic acid so complex as ours to defend
itself against a short, simple nucleic acid like a bacterium.
But in fact the defence has to be very subtle. Our organisation is huge and complicated, containing items as different as
a liver cell and a brain cell. In addition, there are special
cells whose job is simply to circulate round the whole organism clearing up messes, repairing damage, and carrying off
cells that have died or become dangerous in some way. So
we have cells whose sole job is to demolish the chemical
structure created by a nucleic acid exactly the same, to the
last one in millions and millions of subunits, as their own. Yet
we wish to defend this system against the entry of any rival
nucleic acid intent on demolishing it. The basic problem of
defence at this level is therefore one of recognition; and it is
far more difficult than that posed to the radar of a modern
anti-ballistic missile system, which has to choose merely between dummies and real warheads from a multiple-targeted
intercontinental rocket.

Immunology, or the science of self, is the study of this defence system, first because it studies how the self—any individual collection of cells characterised by identical nucleic
acid—defends its organisation against rival nucleic acids.
But second, and much more important, because we have now
discovered that the basic mechanism for solving this problem of recognition is that our nucleic acids define their own
territory by an extremely careful, subtle labelling of all parts
of "self" and an immediate, organised rejection and destruction of anything that is "not-self."

The discovery that self exists in physical terms at the

molecular level and the discovery of how the "selfish" mechanisms work are the essence of modern immunology. Clearly this is a major discovery for both our own body mechanisms and our health. Phrases such as "self-preservation" and "self-determination" now mean something at the cellular level. And immunology has a good deal to say about a wide variety of disease states from the common cold to cancer.

The science of self is called immunology because it arose from the study of mankind's first conscious, brain-directed attempts to repel the competition of rival nucleic acid groups, to make himself immune to some rival.

Presumably man has always been aware of disease. Only for the last twenty years have we been able to see disease as an attempt by rival nucleic acids to take over the chemicals from our own nucleic acids. But for hundreds of years before that men had been consciously, if empirically, warding off rival nucleic acids by immunisation. Immunisation became scientific just over a hundred years ago, when Pasteur discovered the existence of bacteria—or germs—and propounded the germ theory of disease. By luck, as will be related more fully later, he also found out how to help the body defend itself against these germs by immunisation, and in so doing confirmed the validity of the practice of smallpox vaccination, which had been known for centuries.

In a sense immunology is the first of the medical sciences, the first application of the scientific method to curing any of the ills of the body after the discovery of the broad principles by which our bodies work anatomically. It was Pasteur who founded the science of immunology, just as he founded bacteriology and, more important, introduced the methods of science into medicine.

John Maynard Smith, in his book *The Theory of Evolution*,[1] suggests that the most important difference between ourselves and our ancestors of ten thousand years ago that has been brought about by genetic evolution may well be a greater resistance to infectious diseases. Pasteur and his followers in fifty years did more than ten thousand years of evolution by enabling us to provide ourselves with artificial resistance to many of the infectious diseases. This was almost certainly the most important step that has ever been taken in the competition between one set of nucleic acids and the others.

However, in the days when this step was taken it was impossible to see it in this light. The ancient Chinese and Arabs had discovered the technique of smallpox prevention. Pasteur's achievement was to discover the existence of microorganisms, to realise that the "germ" theory accounted for the success of immunisation against smallpox, and then to apply the same technique to other diseases on the basis of this knowledge. The scientific discovery of immunity (as opposed to the uncomprehending practice of it) and the development of a series of useful and life-saving artificial immunities were the start of immunology.

This enormously important and humane field of work remained the main concern of immunology and immunologists until just about twenty years ago. A major step was the discovery of antibodies, the chemicals produced by the animal body specifically to counteract an invading organism or substance. It was understood that the mechanism of artificial immunity was that it stimulated the production of antibodies. These would then be ready in large numbers to defend the body against a really aggressive, virulent invader related to and similar to the weaker "killed" germs administered in the vaccination or inoculation. (In Chapter 4 there will be a more detailed history of this process.)

After its first burst of activity, which ran until about the time of the First World War, immunology remained a rather pedestrian affair for nearly forty years. Few first-class scientists were attracted to it. And the major figures who did work in the field were perhaps mostly chemists or biochemists who studied antibodies and their like primarily from the chemical or biochemical point of view. In the late 1940's many people felt that immunology, once so useful, had come to the end of its career, for the antibiotics had arrived and it seemed that infectious diseases would be wiped out or at least never allowed to get any hold again. People therefore began to turn their attention to those aspects of bodily illness that manifestly were not infectious.

Then suddenly, in the five years 1950 to 1955, modern immunology was born. It was essentially a new science, the science of self, comprehending and absorbing the older immunology—the production of artificial immunities against infectious diseases—from which it grew. A great burst of discovery has continued from 1955 right up to the present day, and still there are many obvious, fundamental questions to be asked in immunology. In laboratories all over the world teams of immunologists are working to get the answers. They are excited, they are invigorating to be among, they all seem to welcome an opportunity to talk about their work. The atmosphere is similar to that which prevailed in nuclear physics thirty years ago.

The change in immunology has been well summed up by Dr. John Humphrey, head of the division of immunology at the National Institute for Medical Research at Mill Hill, a suburb in north London. He is also deputy director of the Institute, which is the largest and most prestigious medical research establishment in Britain despite the fact that it is housed in one of the least attractive buildings designed in the last fifty years. Dr. Humphrey writes in the 1969 *Annual Report* of the Medical Research Council (a feature of the Council *Reports* is that every year four or six subjects are reviewed by one of the best authorities on the subject):

Twenty-five years ago the main and almost sole raison d'être of immunology was the study of immunity against infectious diseases, carried out mostly in departments of bacteriology or pathology. Today, although protection against infectious disease remains a very important aspect of their collective endeavour, immunologists are also to be found in departments of biochemistry, molecular biology, cell biology, dermatology, genetics, haematology, medicine, surgery, and zoology and even in departments styled simply "immunology." Their field of research may be broadly defined as the study of the specific responses of the body to the introduction of foreign materials, or—as Sir Macfarlane Burnet has put it—of the distinction by the body between "self" and "not self." . . . The subject has come to be considered virtually as a discipline in its own right, and it now accounts for a considerable part of the Council's research endeavour.

The idea of immunology as the science of self was the turning point, the start of modern immunology. It arose out of the older style of study that was the speciality of Sir Macfarlane Burnet, an Australian, undoubtedly the most influential scientist that his country has produced, perhaps as important a figure as Rutherford, the New Zealander, had been forty years before him. In essence Burnet's idea emerged from considering the role of immunity against infectious disease as an evolutionary phenomenon. He concluded that the only way in which the animal body could possibly cope with the enormous range of disease organisms threatening it was by some mechanism that recognized what was its "self" and rejected everything else as "not-self." There must be, in fact, on every cell in the world (and, indeed, even on the covering of non-cellular viruses) some sort of "flag" or identification mark. This flag is an expression of the nature of the nucleic acid inside the cell. My body knows its own flag as signifying my self; all other flags indicate not-self to me. But my flag indicates not-self to your body, and likewise to every lion and zebra as well. Your body and mine, the lion's body and the zebra's, can all recognise as not-self the flags on a tubercule bacillus or a measles virus.

When our bodies defend themselves, for instance, by proving immune against a second attack of measles, they show, not that we have learnt from the first attack, but that we have always had inside us a few cells that can specifically attack the measles virus and are designed to do nothing else. The first attack of measles brings these cells into action. They develop, multiply, and produce large quantities of the substance called antibody, which specifically attacks the measles virus. Eventually we recover from the first attack of measles. But ever afterwards we have large numbers of "antimeasles" cells and large quantities of antibody against measles. Thus we can repel all later attacks by the measles virus very quickly—we are, in fact, immune to measles. This corollary to the theory of recognition of self and not-self is known as Burnet's clonal theory and will be explained more fully later on. Burnet has had many other fruitful ideas, but their fuller development fits into the story of immunology at a later stage and belongs in Chapter 5.

Burnet's theory that immunology is the science of self first came out in 1949–50. Within four years, his approach to the problems of immunology had been put onto a firm experimental footing by a team in London, led by Medawar (now Sir Peter Medawar, director of the National Institute for Medical Research). What he proved was that mice could be made to accept skin grafts from other mice if the recipients had been injected with cells from the donor before they were born. This could be interpreted as confirming the idea that a body learns before birth to tolerate, or accept, all those cells which it encounters prenatally, and that those cells are normally only its own. The detail of this work will fill most of a later chapter in this book. For the moment it is sufficient to repeat that Medawar's work put Burnet's ideas onto a sound experimental footing.

A scientific theory is never finally proved true, though it may well be proved untrue. The rejection of the idea that scientific truth comes from observations impartially piling up until a hypothesis presents itself, then to be checked by a well-designed experiment, has been strongly supported by Sir Peter Medawar in his role as philosopher. He upholds the "hypothetico-deductive" model of scientific thought and progress, which has been formally presented by Sir Karl Popper. This approach evaluates a scientific theory in terms of its "testability." It is not so much a question of whether the theory stands up to experimental tests as whether it will provoke tests that produce significant new knowledge. By these standards we cannot say that Medawar's experiments demonstrating the existence of "tolerance" (that is, the ability of one organism to accept cells from another organism or of another type) proved the correctness of Burnet's theory. In many senses it is still not proved true. But Medawar's experiments showed that Burnet's theory was fruitful; it provoked worthwhile and significant advances in knowledge in the ideas it produced and from the experiments done by others to test it.

The introduction of a little philosophy here is not a meaningless digression. Much more will be said, later on, of the effects of Medawar's experiments on philosophical thinking about science. But the important point here is that men of the intellectual stature and wide interests of Macfarlane Burnet and Medawar were now involved in immunology. By the same token, immunology was now concerning itself with ideas and theories that were intellectually exciting.

Science is subject to fashion, like most other human activities. Once a "good man," a brilliant and original research mind, gets going on a particular subject, the brightest students will be attracted to work with him, and other scientists in slightly different fields will be influenced by his ideas and will redirect their work in terms that relate to his ideas and theories. This has been true of immunology. Medawar and Burnet were jointly awarded a Nobel Prize. Both became directors of the largest medical research institutes in their respective countries. Their pupils and the young collaborators of their early days are now professors with departments of their own. But, what is more important, immunology has become even more "fashionable" and exciting, and the ideas these two men started going in the early 1950's are still proving fruitful. Significant discoveries about the mechanism of self-recognition have been made within the last year. There are still big questions implicit in the original ideas that have not been answered, such as how the cells of a body remember the identity of an invader so that they can meet a second aggression by the same invader with better defences. And there are many distinguished scientists in departments of immunology around the world who are thinking up new experiments that they hope will solve these problems.

But immunology as the science of self was also given intellectual stature by being phrased in these terms. For all practical purposes the immunologist cannot see the structures and complexes he is dealing with. Like the chemist, he must demonstrate what is happening chiefly by its effects on much larger organisms than the ones he is interested in. Changes in the reactions of mice or human beings are usually necessary to demonstrate the operation of antibodies, which are molecules of such a size that they can only just be distinguished in electron micrographs—that is, by using the electron microscope.

The intellectually demanding nature of immunology is one of its attractions for many of the most important scientific figures in the field. It is very much a "scientist's science," an arena in which the big men recognise each other as true professionals even where they dislike each other personally. And it is common in scientific disciplines where this feeling of professional superiority reigns to find a substructure within the discipline which is more important to its members than the formal outward structure of university departments and the annual meetings of the specialist society. (Theoretical astronomy is another good example of a scientific discipline where this exists.) The essence of the substructure is that there is a sort of "top table" of "the men who really count": a group of perhaps a couple hundred of men, all of whom know each other personally, and who form a unit quite independent of national boundaries or university structures. Ideas are shuttled about within this group by letters, transatlantic telephone calls, or personal meetings at small symposia, or by exchanging post-doctoral students. These ideas are usually accepted or rejected long before the experimental results which support or tell against them have achieved publication in even the most specialist scientific journals. As one immunologist put it to me: "There are probably five or six thousand scientists round the world who are working in immunology, but there's only two or three hundred who are the real immunologists." (Of course he considered himself, with full justification, one of the select three hundred.)

People who are not scientists too often ignore the fact that scientists are human. There are as many snobs, as many lovers of Beethoven, Shakespeare, and Duke Ellington, as many ambitious men, and as many good cooks among scientists as there are among men of any other profession. From personal and quite unscientific observation, the only exception I can find to this general rule is that an unduly high proportion of the mathematician/physicist class are good piano players. (And there is a distinguished neurophysiologist who has invented the world's only logical bassoon.) The chief, and most important, thing that distinguishes the scientist from other members of society is that almost all scientists are so because they enjoy doing science. Their ambition is nearly always to be known for a piece of good science. They want, of course, the rewards which the world has to offer; but they are not doing that particular job because they want to make a million, because they want power, because they hope to become President, or because they want to become famous. They do science because they like doing it, because usually it appeals to them intellectually or morally.

Failure to realize this quite simple fact about the motivation of most scientists will endanger many of the plans now being made by governments and industries in so many Western countries for the redeployment of scientific effort. You cannot just retrain a biochemist or physicist in order to shift him to the pollution control program; you have to interest him in some scientific problem that arises in pollution control. A clear example of this failure to understand scientific motivation was seen in the troubles experienced by NASA when the moment came for decisions about the objectives of the lunar landing program, after the first successful landing had been achieved. Equally, the fact that scientists do their work for the love of it should not be translated into the hack image of dedicated men selflessly spending their lives in the pursuit of useful knowledge. On the contrary, the motivation of scientists is rather selfish. It is not necessary to enter into moral evaluations. It is simply useful to understand the motivation, so that a due awareness of the scientist's set of worldly values can be reached—why he seems guilty of intellectual snobbery, and why he so values the accolade of "priority," of being the first to suggest or establish something.

In immunology the emergence of the idea of a science of

self, which is obviously a theory of basic importance to one's whole view of "Nature," meant that an enormous area of thought and work was immediately opened up. So basic an idea was applicable in many fields that had previously appeared distinct. It was as though a whole empty continent had been opened up to scientific conquistadores. Into these wide open spaces they flocked, and are still flocking.

At the same time as the basic idea of the science of self was being established, there was of course the parallel establishment of the discipline of molecular biology, with its great opening triumph of the discovery of the mechanism and role of the nucleic acids. There has been no direct link-up yet between these two sciences; at least not in the sense of an explanation of any immunological phenomenon giving a direct demonstration of a change in the order of nucleic acid subunits. But immunology has certainly benefited enormously by the postulation of a mechanism which accounts in comprehensible terms for the observed facts of heredity, and which provides a molecular, or purely chemical explanation for individuality. And the general spread, throughout the disciplines of chemistry and biochemistry, of the notion that the "shape," in three dimensions, of molecules, large and small, accounted for much of their behavior has undoubtedly helped both in the acceptance and the explanation of immunological ideas.

Whether it is a coincidence or an irony that the first important experiments in the new immunology were experiments in transplantation, only the historian will eventually be able to discuss profitably. Transplantation surgery, that most dramatic, most publicised, of recent medical advances, certainly owes its origin to immunology, its greatest problems are immunological ones, and its continuation as an ever more important feature of medical care depends almost solely on the solution by immunologists of these problems. If the immunologists fail here to provide a practical answer to the problems of transplantation (and at least a few of them fear that they may so fail), the moral, ethical, and legal problems that arise from transplantation may never become a serious public issue. For, as every newspaper reader must know, the chief problem in transplantation of most of the major organs of the human body lies in controlling the rejection by the host/recipient of the "foreign" or not-self tissues of the donor.

This is not meant to imply that Medawar invented the idea of transplantation. His experiments were essentially immunological, and used transplantation as a method of questioning a body's reaction to the presence of not-self. But by showing that "tolerance" of not-self could be achieved, he opened people's minds to the possibility of achieving tolerance in a host by several different methods—and this of course meant considering the possibility of transplantation as a standard method of medical treatment where organs had failed. The induction of tolerance in fully grown adults, at the moment as a research project but with an eye to its eventual use in transplant operations, continues to be one of the main lines of immunological research. This research, just as Medawar's before it, will have enormous significance both for the theories of immunity and for the practical results that may spring from it. This is just one example of the wide-open continent of immunological exploration which the concept of a science of self has provided.

The production of tolerance to grafts (or to infection, if for some reason we ever wished to do so) is a matter of manipulating our self-defence, or applying "self-control," if a half-pun can be allowed. But the theory of self and not-self implies more questions and possibilities than this alone. If, for instance, cancer is a display of our own body's cells getting out of control, then surely a cancer cell might be different enough from a normal cell for the body's self-recognising mechanism to spot it and destroy it? Just so, the immunologist will reply, and there is much support for another theory put forward by Sir Macfarlane Burnet, which proposes that throughout its life the human or animal body produces potential cancer cells—cells which have perhaps not copied the nucleic acid correctly from the parent cell—and that these cells are regularly recognized and destroyed. Only the occasional one escapes the normal screening mechanism and is able to set up a colony of dangerous cells descended from itself, which we subsequently recognise as a tumour.

So here again is an immense field for scientific enquiry and activity, which could well have enormous theoretical and practical importance. A number of the most distinguished immunologists are becoming increasingly interested in the connections between cancer and immunology. One obvious line where progress might be made is in an attempt to "ginger up" the defensive forces and self-recognising mechanisms so that they could deal with already established tumours, as well as normally catching potential tumour-forming cells right at the start.

Another question which can be asked is, Does the self-recognising mechanism, as well as occasionally failing, ever go quite wrong, letting loose the defence mechanisms against perfectly normal cells of our own? From this question (and I emphasise that it is the job of a good theory to provoke interesting questions rather than to achieve the impossibility of being proved right) arises the concept of auto-immune disease. Auto-antibodies—antibodies against the producer's own cells—had been discovered before the seminal days of Burnet and Medawar (the discovery dates from 1945; place, London; workers, R. R. A. Coombs, A. E. Mourant, and R. R. Race). They were found in a very obscure, little understood form of anemia and did not fit into any theory or scheme of things until the science of self provided a possible explanation of their existence.

The problems of auto-immune disease, which began as a concept only in 1956 following work by Ivan Roitt and Deborah Doniach at the Middlesex Hospital in London, are many and the answers available so far are distinctly confusing. But the most common of the auto-immune diseases is rheumatoid arthritis, and any work which helps towards the relief of rheumatoid arthritis is bound to be important. Thyroid diseases, certain forms of anemia, some forms of kidney disease, and ulcerative colitis are all believed either to be auto-immune diseases or at least to involve auto-immune phenomena.

Tied in with auto-immune diseases are the problems of allergy. Hay fever is the allergy that most of us know best. But the little itching spot caused by the bite of a comparatively harmless insect like a midge or gnat has likewise turned out to be in the province of the immunologist. So have farmer's lung, asthma, and the cotton spinners' disease, byssinosis. The common factor in all these diseases, and the reason the immunologist is involved with them as well as with insect bites, is that the root cause of the trouble is the invasion of the body by foreign substances—the insects' saliva, the pollen grains from grasses, the moulds and mites of house dust, and the plant products of cotton. The reaction of the body's immune system in these cases is exaggerated, the sufferers from these diseases are hypersensitive, and an unwanted antibody is probably participating. Even if he does not produce cures in a dramatically short time, there is more work here for the immunologist: to provide some explanation linking these previously rather inexplicable troubles is something of a triumph for the science of self.

Again, if the body is organised to reject any cell, or even substance, which is not itself, how are we to account for a mother carrying a baby in her womb? The baby receives at least half its nucleic acid from its father, which means the mother's body should certainly reject it as not being herself. We know, of course, that the mother does not reject her infant; and she even gives it some of her own immunity to infectious diseases to protect her infant during the first months of life outside the womb, until the infant can develop its own defensive mechanisms.

The questions posed by the concept of a self-recognising system go on and on, and most of them seem to have this fascinating property of being both intellectually interesting and likely to lead to valuable practical results. Pursuing the thoughts about mother and child, for instance, why does not the woman reject the man's sperm before conception occurs? Or, alternatively, could we immunise a woman against her husband's cells (or, for that matter, against any man's sperm) and so achieve contraception through immunological means?

The question, Why does a mother not reject her child? prompts an opposite idea—Why does a child not reject its mother? The answer is undoubtedly that a foetus in the womb is incapable of immune reactions—the defence mechanisms only develop activity after birth—it was by exploiting this fact that Medawar was able to show the existence of tolerance. But we can ask an analogous question: Why does not a graft damage the recipient? The graft may well contain part of the donor body's defensive system still in working order, and this should react against the recipient. So, in fact, it does; and the immunologist has to comprehend what is known as "graft-versus-host" reaction.

The science of self, then, has illuminated a wide variety of dark corners, and may well help to solve a large number of problems. But like most human activities, it probably raises as many problems as it solves—we can already see something of the legal and ethical problems that real achievement in transplantation surgery may raise. There is a pleasant irony in the fact that the circle is now round almost to the starting point.

The arrival of the antibiotics, in many senses, forced the older immunology to turn in on itself and seek theories to account for its many earlier successes against disease. The antibiotics seemed to promise the virtual ending of infectious disease, and immunologists, like other men, want to keep their jobs in existence. Perhaps this expresses the historical situation rather crudely; however, several of the older immunologists have described a feeling akin to this as leading them to take certain jobs at the end of the Second World War, jobs that led them to their present eminence as theoretical immunology opened up. Now we are disillusioned about the ability of the antibiotics to control all infectious diseases. Bacteria develop resistance to antibiotics; and insects, for that matter, have developed resistance to DDT and similar insecticides that we had hoped would kill off the insect transmitters of many tropical diseases. Further, antibiotics are almost powerless against viruses (though very recently there has appeared one antibiotic, rifampicin, that has hopeful anti-viral properties). So now we are again turning to the immunologists' approach to lead the fight against infectious diseases.

This brings the immunologist up against such difficult problems as the control of influenza and the common cold. Influenza is tricky because the virus seems to be able to change its external appearance quite rapidly, thus deceiving the immune system, which has been activated (by inoculation or by previous infection) to recognise the virus in an earlier shape. The common cold seems to be caused by no fewer than eighty different types of virus, and preparing vaccine against that number of aggressors seems impossible.

Then there is malaria, probably the greatest cause of ill-health in tropical countries; malaria seems to break most of the rules of immunity to which we are accustomed. Nevertheless, most of the oddities observed, or suspected, in malarial infections fit reasonably well into a picture based on the self-recognition system, at least when that system is overwhelmed. So the immunologist must try to deal with infectious diseases more difficult, though perhaps often less lethal, than the ones that faced his predecessors. But now he has the benefit of a reasonable conceptual basis on which to form his ideas for research into the new subject.

To sum up so far: the science of self, the concept that all higher creatures have a system of recognising their self material and of rejecting not-self, has not only proved extremely useful in combating disease and starting new approaches to practical problems in medicine; it has also proved an extremely fruitful and stimulating idea. A scientific discipline has been founded on the basis of this concept, combined with the technology of dealing with infectious diseases by immunological methods. The pursuit of the many questions and implications inherent in the original concept forms the most exciting of the sciences at the moment.

It was an immunologist, Sir Peter Medawar, who said, "Ideas are the lifeblood of science. They can't be bought; they can sometimes be sold."

Chapter 2

The Importance of Knowing Who You Are

"Self" is a word which we almost always use in a humane context, and a concept we normally associate with psychological studies. It is also a very emotional word.

Combine "self" with one set of words—self-pity, self-importance, self-righteousness, self-deception—and you get a set of ideas which comes very low in our scale of values, probably right at the bottom. Combine "self" with another set of words—self-determination, self-control, self-defense—and there is a set of concepts of which we approve. The great religions of the world place yet another set of meanings on "self" and its combinations. From Buddhism to Christianity they preach that we must abandon self if we seek happiness and salvation. "Self-denial" is a virtue to be practised, with special seasons set aside for extra effort. "Self-sacrifice" is the noblest of all actions.

But the concept of "self" as it is used in this book is just as valid as the humane concept. It may be more mechanical, more deterministic, but all the other concepts of "self" depend on this one—the concept of "self" as a bodily self; "self" as the physical definition of the body of an individual. If I look at my skin, I can see with my eyes a boundary between "myself" and the rest of the universe. One side of this boundary is "me," the other side is "not-me." When a scientist looks more closely at that boundary he sees that the skin cells are dead, that atoms are shooting out of "me" all the time and other atoms shooting into "me." There is no absolute line of demarcation between "me" and the rest of the universe. I must define my "self" (myself) as those atoms which are part of the system organised by my nucleic acid.

The scientific use of the word "self" must carry none of the emotional overtones of the humane word. It means nothing but the ability of an organism to recognise those cells and biological products which are its own parts. All organisms, from the simplest amoeba upwards, have some "self" defence, but specific "self"-recognition is a feature only of the higher organisms—the vertebrates, the creatures from fish through reptiles, to birds, mammals, and men which have bony spines. To any of these organisms, "self" is divided simply from "not-self," and "not-self" means the rest of the universe. "Self" in the scientific sense is a matter of molecular chemistry.

"Self" must not be confused with "individuality." The self-recognition mechanism of any organism is assumed to lie in a particular sequence of subunits of the nucleic acids which are in every cell of that organism—or perhaps in several different sequences. No one knows what those sequences are, or even where they lie on the acid chains. But in identical twins, two creatures derived from a single conception, the nucleic acids are identical. Therefore, the self-recognition sequences are identical; therefore, each twin recognises tissues from the other as its own. In practice, this means that grafts between identical twins are not rejected. But no one denies that those two creatures, twin calves or twin humans, are separate individuals.

They are different individuals in time; that is to say that

many things do not occur to them or affect them simultaneously. They are different individuals in space; above all, they have different memories. To the scientist, who by definition cannot observe the individual soul or spirit, the firmest reason for believing in the completely separate individuality of human beings is that each one must have different memories. Theoretically, at least, these different memories, whether they be chemical changes or patterns of electrical circuits in the brain cells, should be observable.

It is well known now that there are other human beings whose sequence of self-recognition subunits is so similar to mine that a graft of an organ from them to me has a better-than-average chance of not being rejected immediately. (This is the basis of tissue typing or tissue matching, which will come more fully into the picture later on.) It is just conceivable that by some virtually incalculable chance there might be some other human quite unrelated to me, whose entire nucleic acid has exactly the same order of subunits as mine, but because we have lived different lives at slightly different times, the different memories would provide a scientific method of distinguishing between us.

The thought that one's self is no more than a mechanism for defence against infectious disease or cancer, that one's individuality lies in nothing but memory, that one's life is only a device of spiral molecules for preserving themselves and passing themselves on to future generations, is probably inexpressibly dreary for most people. I remember discussing this in a BBC Third Programme broadcast with John Watkins, of the London School of Economics, a philosopher of Sir Karl Popper's persuasion, and with Sir Peter Medawar. Medawar made the point, which I now wish to emphasise, that this is not a *whole* view of life; it is simply the appearance of some of life's mechanisms as seen from one biological viewpoint. From exactly the same viewpoint, the intermingling of all the genetic factors that play a part in controlling and determining personality, the enormous variation among individuals, is a far grander concept than any of those founded simply on the preservation of the individual. As Medawar said then, people enjoy life, and furthermore we participate in the process as individuals. When a teacher finds that something he has taught is growing in the minds of others, he has made a personal impact upon the genetic flux that goes on through generation after generation.

Looking at life from this biological viewpoint also ignores the evolution of culture and tradition, knowledge and know-how—what Medawar calls the "exogenetic" evolution. Because it is not seen from this particular viewpoint does not mean that even the most dedicated immunologist regards these things as nonexistent or insignificant. Cultural evolution is acknowledged by all as the peculiarly human contribution: if, for the rest of this book, it is virtually ignored, that is simply because it is not observable at the cellular or molecular level.

In any case I cannot think it irrelevant that the problem of self and individual identity is so much in the minds of the artists, writers, philosophers, and playwrights of today, just as it is in the minds of the scientists. The great artist must surely be a prophet (in the biblical sense) as well as an entertainer. The plays of Pinter, Beckett, and Ionesco are concerned, among other things, with the isolation of individuals, with the inability to break through the barriers of the humane self by communication. "Who am I?" is a question often asked in twentieth-century literature, however it may be phrased. Saul Bellow, for instance, asked it in *Dangling Man* in 1944, just when immunologists were starting on the work that would bring them to ask a similar question scientifically. Ten years later, as the immunologists were putting the question openly, Nigel Dennis was writing a fantasia on the same subject called *Cards of Identity*. From the Renaissance and the Reformation to this side of the French Revolution, the main drive of Western history can be seen as a drive for individual freedom. But in the twentieth century, revolutions are not made for individual freedom—neither the Russian, the Chinese, nor the Cuban revolutions has aimed at individual freedom. And in the non-Communist countries it is no longer reactionary or illiberal to think of limiting individual freedoms for the sake of the good of the community. If the thinking of our culture is nowadays dominated by the "crisis of the individual," there is a parallel trend in science. Immunology, the science of self, may help to provide a cool and reasonably firm foundation upon which to erect the mental structures of the next stage in our cultural evolution.

The physical existence of the concept of "self" seems to have arisen at the stage of evolution which is marked by such creatures as the lamprey, the hagfish, and the lemon basking shark. This is not to say that creatures "lower" in the evolutionary order do not have defences against aggressors; plainly they do have some mechanism for preserving the integrity of their organisms and of the nucleic acid inside. An amoeba, the simplest of single-cell creatures, can both resist a bacterium and refrain from digesting itself. There is really no answer to any question about *how* this is managed. But whatever the defences of the lower creatures, including the insects and plants, may be, it is clear that they are not specific mechanisms; that is to say, they may react to an invader but this is probably only a reaction against invasion, not against that particular invader. Further, they have apparently no greater immunity after one attack to a further aggression by that same attacker. Their response is "nonspecific."

The fruiting wood of one type of apple can be grafted

onto the root stock of another type; this is the basis of much modern scientific fruit farming. But one hagfish can be grafted onto another and the rejection, if any, will be very slow. It is only the vertebrates that reject skin grafts, only the vertebrates that defend themselves against an attack of smallpox with different chemicals than they normally defend themselves against cholera and in such a way that after one attack they are immune, or prepared, against further attacks. The vertebrates possess a system of specific adaptive immunity, a system which specifically recognises itself and equally can distinguish to a considerable degree of fineness between varieties of not-self. It can adapt its own mechanisms so that having once met a specific type of not-self, it is more efficient in dealing with that type of not-self in the future.

This sort of immunity is believed to have started developing in evolutionary terms at the level of the hagfish and the lamprey: both parasites, both in the class of cyclostomes, the predecessors of the true fishes. A hagfish will get right in among the muscle of the fish it is parasitising, dissolving the muscle and killing the fish. The lamprey only attaches itself to the fish it is parasitising and sucks its blood. A hagfish can for all practical purposes be grafted onto another hagfish. A lamprey has a primitive immune system and will slowly recognise a piece of skin from another lamprey grafted onto it and reject it. Lampreys might be considered very powerful evolutionary forces if they meet a population unprepared for them. At one time lampreys were confined to Lake Ontario, but when the Welland Canal was cut to bypass Niagara Falls, the lampreys came through the canal and in a few years had virtually wiped out the trout of Lake Superior and the other Great Lakes.

So one suggestion, and it is no more than a suggestion, as to how the mechanism of adaptive immune self-recognition came about is that in Silurian times the primitive lampreys, which were among the first of the vertebrates, were parasitising their own kind, perhaps the young parasitising their own parents. This set up enormous evolutionary pressure to "find an answer" to the threat. One answer was to grow bony skins over the stomach and other visceral organs. This type of creature, the ostracoderm, died out. The other answer was to develop a mechanism for recognising not-self, even when the particular type of not-self was closely related to the self, and then be able to reject the not-self.

The essence of self is a chain of nucleic acid which has its subunits in a different order from that of any other creature, even if at the extreme this means that only one subunit among the thousands or millions is different from the nearest related creature. But the hereditary nucleic acids are kept mostly in the nucleus, a sort of central bag within the main bag of the cell. They do not come into contact with the nucleic acids of other cells in the normal course of living. Therefore, a self-recognition system must embody some expression on the surface of the cell of the type of nucleic acid that lies within the nucleus. Nobody knows exactly what form this expression takes, but we are pretty sure it is there. We call it the antigen, and there is good reason to believe that its most essential feature is its shape. Over-simplifying for the moment, there must be either knobs or holes on the surface of every cell and the knobs or holes on the surfaces of my cells are different from those on yours. The suggestion is that this is the sort of system which the primitive lampreys evolved in order to deal with parasitisation by their own kind. All this, and what immediately follows, is Sir Macfarlane Burnet's elaboration of his original theory over the years.

This mechanism demands more than just the setting up of "self-markers," like little personal flags flying on the surface of every cell you own. It demands the setting up of a group of cells whose primary task is to circulate around the body examining everything they come across for their self or not-self flags. One of the big excitements among immunologists today is the argument over whether more than one type of cell has been allotted this task. At this writing, there are many experiments afoot designed to answer just this question. But it is widely accepted that a system of cells, the immune cells, must have been set up and must be with us now, to do this job. Most immunologists now agree in believing these are the white cells called lymphocytes.

How do the immune cells learn to recognise self and not-self cells? What do they do when they meet a not-self cell? How does the body reject a cell identified as not-self? The answers, I hope, or at least the tentative answers that immunologists are giving at the moment, will come in the course of the rest of this book. The point to make here is that since this system can, by the time it has reached our stage of evolution, cope with every different type of not-self from a measles virus to a tapeworm parasite to an organ grafted from another human being by twentieth-century surgeons, an enormous range of variation must have become built into it. This means that at some stage both in evolution as a whole and in each individual life ("ontogeny" is the scientific term), the genetic material must have to produce a number of cells, broadly of the same type, but with many minor variations so that they can in some way recognise the antigens on the cells of worms and germs and advanced mammals. This implies a lability in cells of this sort: instead of simply copying the parent cell time and time again, with at most some comparatively slow differentiation into liver cells or brain cells, considerable variety, at least in surface features, must be produced in a short time.

This is where the origin of cancer may be found, at least in an evolutionary sense. Cancer is not an invader from out-

side, it is not an infectious or contagious disease. It is a variation from true breeding in one of our own cells. We know in
our own time that this variation from true breeding can be
caused by external forces, by radiation, by viruses (at least
in birds and animals, though it has never yet been conclusively proved in a human sufferer), by cigarette smoking, by
inhaling asbestos dust, and by many other agents. But there
are also many "spontaneous" tumours in which no outside influence can be incriminated. In these cases there is, apparently, again some lability in the genetic mechanism, which
allows the production of a cell that has not accurately repro-
duced the nucleic acid from the parent cell. The faulty nucleic acid (probably) allows both the movement and the
reproduction rate of the aberrant cell to avoid the normal
control exerted on it (probably, again) by the adjacent cells.

Although there have recently been experiments which
have produced something very like cancer in plants, on the
whole cancer is a peculiarity of vertebrates. It is not unreasonable to believe that it may, then, have arisen at the same
time in evolution as the vertebrates, and the simultaneous
development of a lability in cell mechanisms might well be
the reason for this. The story seems to be reasonable, though
there is really almost nothing available in the way of proof.
If, however, cancers did arise at the same time, they would
simply put more evolutionary pressure in favor of the rapid
development of an immune system which could screen them
out and destroy them before they could become founders of
a tumour consisting of their own progeny. We know that
cancer cells do present some antigenic surfaces, and it is not
unreasonable to suppose that these may very well be of the
not-self kind. Certainly the body can make antibodies
against some types of cancer cell.

It must be said, however, that we know just as little about
the evolution of bacteria and viruses. Because they have no

bony structure, they have left no fossil traces. As they are simple organisms it is reasonable to assume that they developed early in evolutionary history—but this is not necessarily so. The same non-picture exists for worms and other parasites. But today the specific adaptive immune system of the vertebrates operates against bacteria, viruses, and parasites of the worm type; and it operates by spotting them as not-self and organising the machinery for their specific destruction, type by type. In turn, many of these rival groups of nucleic acids have developed mechanisms by which they can avoid the attentions of the immune systems of the bigger organisms. Some worms seem to have the ability to "disguise" themselves with something very like the host body's "self-marker" antigens. Some bacteria and viruses seem to be able to live comfortably within a host for years, or even, when inside the intestinal tract, to live as an ally of the host throughout its life. The influenza virus has a different trick. It has apparently developed a lability of the genetic mechanism, much as has been suggested in the theory of the evolution of cancer, so that it can develop new strains with different antigens fairly frequently, thus depriving the host of the advantage of having "learnt" the shape of the influenza antigens in some previous experience of invasion. It is just as likely that we have evolved our immune system, our self-preservation system, as a defence against what we commonly call "germs," as for any other reason.

The essential words here are "our self-preservation system." The essence of this system is that it protects one organism, the individual, against all other organisms. The nucleic acids which both build and define the individual organism, and which are contributed in equal portions by the two different parents, express themselves on the surface of every cell of that organism. The nucleic acid of every individual differs from that of any other individual (except an identical twin) by at least a difference in the order of some of the subunits. And somehow this difference is expressed in a difference on the cell surface. The same nucleic acids also organise a system of cells and activities which have somehow "learnt" to tolerate those cells that present self-antigens, and which yet are able to recognise any other antigen that may invade the organism. In theory they can destroy the invader, the possessor of not-self antigens. Thus the system is in the strict meaning of the word a "self-preservation" system.

The self-preservation system can go wrong in many ways; usually only then do we become aware of it. It can be overcome by an invasion of not-self organisms which is numerically too large for it to cope with, or where the invading organism multiplies itself more rapidly than the defending forces can destroy the invading individuals. Then we say that the animal has died of an infectious disease. The system itself can be weakened by improper functioning of one of its parts; this may well be the case in old age. There are also many types of congenital weakness in the system—children are born with poorly functioning immune systems. The system can be damaged by external forces, such as radiation or chemicals, and these external forces can be intentionally applied for the benefit of the organism as a whole, as in the case of transplant surgery. The immune system is quite incapable of "knowing" whether it acts for the long-term advantage or disadvantage of the whole organism. Likewise, the system can be "deceived" by such invaders as parasites which present antigens sufficiently similar to self-antigens to "put it off its guard."

The system is not infallible. It can over-react, as in the case of allergies. It can under-react, as possibly in the case of cancer cells, when the antigens of the aberrant self cells do not give a clear definition of whether they are self or not-self. And the system can turn against itself, as in the case of auto-immune diseases, where apparently its destructive activities are turned against self cells. There are also cases, such as those of men who produce antibody against their own sperm, where the immune system can act against the interests of the organism as a whole.

As a vertebrate in the twentieth century man has inherited this system. For all practical purposes we can do nothing to change it—although just possibly in the future, when we know a great deal more about the details of its working and if ever genetic engineering becomes a practicable technique, it is conceivable that we might be able to modify it. We have learnt, however, how to help our immune systems, an empirical discovery if ever there was one. But on a real "suck it and see" basis, and without any theoretical understanding of how the system worked, we have practised prophylactic immunisation by which we "primed" our immune systems and activated the defences against specific invaders before the body had met them in the course of nature. This system has not yet been perfected: notably, we cannot protect against the common cold and a number of similar diseases, largely because our immune system works against specific invaders and in these cases a wide variety of different specific invaders appears to cause the same medical condition.

There is some hope that we may be able to help our immune system in a rather different way in dealing with cancer. Here we have either got to increase its activity against cells with "weak" antigens or to improve the subtlety and fine definition of its ability to recognise tumour cells.

Our other immediate prospects of improving our situation in practical medical terms depend mainly on controlling the immune reaction or making it work to our benefit when its automatic response to the situation happens to be disadvantageous to the organism's long-term good. Thus we hope that by suppressing the "immune reaction," we can make transplant surgery into a much more common and useful standard medical treatment for the failure of organs. We could also approach this problem of overcoming the rejection of transplanted organs by inducing tolerance in the host for the antigens of the donor. There are a number of ways in which this might be done, in addition to that by which Medawar and his colleagues achieved it in those first experiments, which had more importance for the theory of immunology than they have yet had for the practice of immunological control.

Hopes of controlling the immune reaction when it has "gone wrong" in the case of auto-immune diseases and allergies depend, at the moment, even more on our reaching a better understanding of the processes. The prospect of immunising women against their husbands' sperm and thus achieving immunological contraception may perhaps be far in the future, for the principles involved seem to be little understood. Again, it would seem to be a case of increasing the immune response rather than controlling it.

This sort of crystal-gazing may seem, at first sight, no better than Sunday supplement journalism. But, with the obvious qualification that all forecasts may be wrong, there are good reasons for spelling out the possible future benefits that may be provided by present-day immunological research.

One reason is that these possible improvements in medical treatment are among the explicit hopes of the men engaged in immunological research. Secondly, an extremely interesting report, entitled *Medicines in the 1990's,* was produced in Britain in 1969 by the Office of Health Economics. This organisation is supported by the pharmaceutical industry, and therefore may be thought to have an obvious axe to grind; nevertheless, it has built up a perfectly sound reputation for its statistical and economic reports. *Medicines in the 1990's* is a piece of technological forecasting: it used the so-

called Delphi technique of forecasting, originally developed
by the Rand Institute in the United States. Many people
scorn technological forecasting, and hold that all its proposals are of little more value than the "hunches" of any well-
informed person. Equally there are those (and I include myself among them) who believe that such techniques do offer
at least a rational guide to those areas in which we can most
profitably direct our efforts. And although doubtless there
will be unexpected developments, it should also be possible
to improve the techniques of sensible forecasting. The
Delphi technique can be described as a controlled form of
"brainstorming," where the obvious imperfections of personality interactions, of undue influence by powerful personali-
ties or over-favorable presentation of a particular viewpoint,
or the tendency to "get on the bandwagon," are all averted
by keeping the participants apart. In the case of the Office of
Health Economics' attempt at medical forecasting, the participants were distinguished, or well qualified, or both, and
represented Holland and Sweden as well as the United States
and Britain. This report, therefore, though it contains some
predictions which seem "sensational," represents the proper
application of a well-known technique of forecasting to the
medical field.

In almost every section of discussion of possible improvements in clinical medical practice the report predicts advances resulting from immunological research now in progress. Dealing with Bacterial Infections, for instance, where
the general conclusion is that "In bacterial infections there
are likely to be many small changes but few big ones over the
next twenty years," the report goes on to suggest, "There will
also be a better understanding of the process of intracellular
survival of bacteria and of the biochemical bases of harmful
hypersensitivity and of auto-immune processes which accompany long term persistence of bacteria and their products in

the tissues. This may affect the therapy of a number of diseases not at present recognised as bacterial in origin." There is, further, a suggestion that vaccines may be developed against the sexually transmitted diseases, and it is pointed out that the effect of these will be as much social as medical.

On virus infections the vaccines that the immunologists will produce (or are even now producing) will obviously have important effects. Measles vaccine is now with us; vaccine against German measles (rubella), with its well-known effects on unborn babies, is coming onto the market even as I am writing. A mumps vaccine is already in use in some countries. Written in late 1969, the report says: "In the case of the viruses causing serum and infective hepatitis [jaundice], the causal agents should have been isolated and cultured during the next five years." In fact, one of these agents seems certainly to have been discovered in the first months of 1970. And if viruses are the causal agents of any human tumours (the report suggests that some such cases may well be identified by 1980), then again vaccines could be helpful. Study is also beginning of the so-called slow virus diseases, which refers to the suspicion that the scrapie disease of sheep, the obscure "kuru" disease known only among the Stone Age inhabitants of New Guinea, and multiple sclerosis in Western countries may all have a similar causative agent, a virus or even a more obscure particle which can lie dormant in a host for years before being stimulated into destructive activity. A more likely target for immunologists and their vaccines are the so-called syncytial viruses which cause bronchitis and other respiratory diseases in young children. These vaccines may be available within ten years.

On immunisation against influenza and the common cold, however, the report is less optimistic; it doubts whether the public can be persuaded to accept the repeated revaccinations that seem likely to be necessary against all the forms of influenza. The possibility of developing an immunisation against all the varieties of viruses that cause common colds seems remote.

Under the headings of Cancer, Graft Rejections, Contraception, and Auto-Immune Diseases, the report on the medicine of the next twenty years makes forecasts broadly in line with those I have already outlined, but it makes them rather more precisely. Thus for instance, it predicts that as early as 1975 there may be the first attempts to make babies born with congenital heart disease tolerant of animal tissues by injecting them with cells from an animal before birth, and then transplanting the heart from the same animal into the human baby.

But the report suggests entirely new prospects for using the results of present immunological research in dealing with heart disease and diseases of the blood vessels (vascular disease). It proposes a wide variety of treatments, based on injecting into the heart tissue-culture extracts containing the buds of capillary (very small) blood vessels to replace those damaged by myocardial infarction (heart attack), and accompanying them with growth-stimulating substances so that surgery to replace damaged arteries and veins will no longer be necessary. Similar treatment and blood vessel grafts will be widely used in the vascular diseases.

In the very different field of disorders of the metabolism and biochemistry of the body, and hormonal disorders, immunology can again help in the future. This time it will be by means of the techniques which the immunologists have developed for their own use for measuring with great accuracy the minute quantities of biochemicals and enzymes they are interested in. These techniques applied to metabolic and hormonal disorders will enable us, possibly during the next ten years, to learn enough about the bases and origins of these disorders to start thinking about controlling them.

Finally, after boldly predicting that the basic research of 1970 to 1980 will enable us in the 1980's to produce substances which will give us control of most allergies, the report points out that technology will steadily be producing even more substances, in the shape of new foods, new medicines, and new inventions, to which we can become allergic.

In an attempt to achieve some form of unity, this chapter has telescoped about 400 million years of evolutionary history and about forty years of the future into some 4,000 words. Warning has duly been given that there is no proof of what has been said about either past or future—it is simply a matter of the best guess on both sides of the present. The only proof of these predictions about the future will come during the remainder of the twentieth century. But it is possible to assemble some of the evidence that makes for the current view of the evolution of an adaptive immunological system in all mammals, birds, and fishes; indeed, in all vertebrates.

So back to the hagfish and the lamprey. The hagfish, as we have seen, is virtually unable to reject a graft from another hagfish; the lamprey will reject a graft, if only slowly. This has been shown in modern laboratory experiments, and the modern hagfish and lamprey are assumed to be representative of similar forms of primitive fish which the fossil record shows to have been the ancestors of more developed fish. Now the hagfish does have a few cells which look very much like the cells we call lymphocytes in modern mammals and men, birds, fishes, and reptiles. For the moment we will leave it that these lymphocytes play a vital part in immunological mechanisms. In the hagfish the lymphocytes appear to play a part in chronic inflammation.

In the next step up the evolutionary ladder, the lampreys, we find true lymphocytes, the first signs of the organ called the thymus, and the first primitive spleen. The thymus is an organ which, like lymphocytes, will occupy much space in later chapters. The spleen is known to have something to do with the immunological mechanisms, but otherwise it shares with the pineal gland the distinction of being an organ whose function, even in modern man, continues to baffle us. With this primitive mechanism the lamprey can not only reject grafts but also produce antibodies and gammaglobulins. And it has an "immune memory," which means that, once it has met an antigen to which it can react, it "remembers" it and reacts much more violently when it meets it for a second time. All these activities are very slow and weak in the lamprey, and when it was tested against twenty known antigens it was able to make antibody against only one—the brucella organism, which causes spontaneous abortion in cows and brucellosis in man.

Further up the evolutionary tree, creatures show more developed immunological systems. The guitarfish has a thymus very similar to a mammal's thymus and has been shown to react to six of the twenty antigens used as tests by Professor Robert Good, who is American Legion Memorial Heart Research Professor of Pediatrics and Microbiology in the Department of Pediatrics at the University of Minnesota Medical School, Minneapolis. "Bob" Good will appear many times in later pages of this book. For seven years now he has had a considerable team, including his wife Dr. Joanne Finstad, working with at least thirty species of fish, amphibians, reptiles, birds, and mammals in an attempt to trace the evolution of immunological mechanisms, following up the suggestions of Macfarlane Burnet and others. The modern representatives of the creatures which arose about 250 million years ago, the higher sharks and the paddlefish, seem to have a complete repertoire of organs associated with immune responses and they make antibodies to all the twenty antigens used as test material. Good writes: "The studies emphasize the fundamental importances of the lymphoid system to the survival of vertebrates. Nature knows a good thing when she sees it and every animal form phylogenetically distal to [i.e., which developed from] the lamprey has a thymus." [1]

But was this system of immune responses evolved primarily to deal with outside invaders—germs, bacteria, and viruses—or was it developed to deal with internal problems? Good lists nine principal relationships or interfaces between malignancies and immunity: (1) All chemicals known to cause cancers also suppress the immune response in patients or experimental animals; (2) all chemicals that suppress the immune response foster cancers even if they do not cause them themselves; (3) experimental procedures, such as removing the thymus, that depress immunological vigour foster the development of malignancy; (4) effective suppression of immune responses in patients (e.g., those who have received transplants) is accompanied by a rapid rise in the incidence of malignancy; (5) diseases of immunological deficiency are associated with the occurrence of malignancies at a far higher rate than in people without such disease; (6) in the case of people who have malignant disease, it is very often possible to show a clear reduction in immunological responses; (7) the incubation period of certain cancers is accompanied by demonstrable defects in immunological function; (8) advanced age is a period of declining immunological vigour, when cancers develop more frequently than among younger people; and (9) once one primary cancer has appeared, other primary cancers are of great frequency (as well as secondary tumours arising from the first primary cancer).

"These findings," declares Professor Good, "seem necessary corollaries of the basic concept that the primary raison d'être for immunologic adaptation is to provide defense against malignant adaptation." He produced these arguments in 1969 at a symposium on cancers in lower animals, and he challenged the symposium to prove him wrong by showing that invertebrates could ever get cancers at all, still less that they get them as often as vertebrates. "We have not yet been satisfied that the lumps and bumps or cellular accumulations among the invertebrates have features that are associated with the malignant tumors of mammals," he said; [2] but his own laboratory had shown that lampreys can have malignancies, and that malignancies similar in character to those of mammals can be found in fishes, reptiles, and amphibia.

Yet another telling set of facts was produced by Professor Good at this symposium: all vertebrates from man through mouse down to lamprey have circulating round cells (lymphocytes and their relatives), which can be easily destroyed by radiation and by chemicals (steroids) of the kind we use to suppress immune reactions. All vertebrates can be killed by radiation in a dose of about 1,000 rads. Invertebrates do not appear to have such cells, and they can also survive doses of radiation ten or one hundred times as high as those which kill a vertebrate.

The hagfish in fact can stand ten times as much radiation as the lamprey; and so in evolution something was lost as well as gained with the coming of the immune system and the development of the lymphoid tissues which house the immune mechanisms. Says Professor Good of "Disorders of the Immune System":

> This suggests that the selective pressures favouring the development of the lymphoid system must have been enormous. I doubt very much that the system originally had anything to do with defenses against infection because, among other things, invertebrates have no such defenses—yet compete successfully with vertebrates in every ecologic niche. My guess is that lymphoid development was definitely connected with

the appearance of more and more elaborate species during the course of evolution, that it reflected the survival value of having improved control over proliferation in increasingly complex tissues among the vertebrates. . . . But you simply cannot have variation and still have genetically stable species. So there had to be a kind of police system which in the event of somatic variation could distinguish "self" from "nonself" cells and destroy the latter. In other words lymphoid mechanisms probably first developed, not to defend against outsiders or outside antigens, but to defend against and eliminate unwanted insiders that "bore from within" and threaten the integrity of the individual and the survival of the species.[3]

So how does the immune system work?

Our General Defences

It would be quite wrong to go ahead with a more detailed description of the specific immune mechanisms of the body without making it very clear that this is not the body's *only* means of defence. There is a wide variety of other defences both internal and external, and in the evolutionary terms of this chapter these non-specific methods of defence must account also for the protection of those very successful life forms, such as plants and insects, which have not developed specific immune mechanisms.

There is first and foremost the skin, the obvious outer defence and covering of the body. The skin is a great deal more than just a covering: it has active anti-bacterial chemicals on and in it, as well as its physical ability to prevent entry. Slightly gruesome experiments have shown this clearly—for instance, if a culture of salmonella typhi, typhoid germs, is smeared on the skin and then regularly sampled every few minutes, it has been found that in twenty minutes the number of living micro-organisms is reduced to very few. Similar samples taken simultaneously from a culture of the germs spread on a glass plate continue, however, to show great activity and large numbers of viable bacteria all the time. A third smear of the germs on the skin of a human corpse behaves much more like the smear on the glass. Chemicals such as lactic acid in the sweat and acids from the sebaceous glands near the roots of hairs are thought to be responsible for this sort of anti-bacterial defence, and it is significant that conditions such as "athlete's foot," which is caused by a fungus type of micro-organism, occur between the toes and on the underside of the foot where there are no hairs. It is probably for the same sort of reason that a cleaning woman's hands and arms, continually sodden with washing water, are likely sites of infection.

A similar type of outer defence against all invaders is provided by the mucus of the nose and genital organs, and the tear-liquid of the eyes. All these can be shown clearly in the laboratory to possess powers of killing bacteria and viruses. Undoubtedly the substance which is attracting most interest nowadays is the enzyme called lysozyme; it is found in human tears and was first characterized by Sir Alexander Fleming, the discoverer of penicillin, as long ago as 1922. Lysozyme has the power of bursting the "skin," more properly the cell wall, of many types of bacteria. It is now suspected of existing in many other places as well as in tears, and this ability to break cell walls may play a part in many other processes. These other activities are not of immediate concern here, beyond pointing out that this powerful substance is part of our outer and general defence system.

When we consider the other obvious entry point into the body, the mouth and the tract down through the stomach to the intestines, we find another simple but strong defence system in that these apparently easy routes of invasion are kept in a condition of such high acidity (primarily in order to break down food for digestive purposes) that few, if any, bacteria can live in them; they are therefore almost completely sterile.

In quite different terms there is also the phenomenon of genetic immunity. What this means in detail, how it works, is really quite unknown. But undoubtedly it is extraordinarily difficult to give a rat diphtheria that will kill it—whereas men and guinea-pigs are easy victims of this organism. There is not much practical use to be made at the moment from this sort of genetic immunity; in fact, it is usually just a difficulty faced by laboratory workers, meaning that they cannot use some particular animal for their research. This has long been a problem in studying leprosy—a germ that has been brought within the reach of many of the normal research techniques only because of the very recent discovery that the mycobacterium which causes leprosy can be grown in the foot-pad of a mouse.

There are some differences of resistance to particular germs even within one species: Algerian sheep are apparently more resistant to anthrax than European sheep. And it has been possible to produce strains of rabbits that are conspicuously either more or less resistant than normal to tuberculosis. This variation of genetic resistance to disease, though very far from being understood, has been notably useful so far only to the plant breeders in providing strains of wheat and rice resistant to rusts and other plant viruses. We cannot, of course, carry out breeding experiments with men and it is almost impossible ever to be certain whether some human races are more resistant to certain diseases than others for genetic reasons or whether the apparent differences in resistance are accidents of history or environment.

In the Second World War, for instance, there were several nasty outbreaks of poliomyelitis among young British

soldiers and sailors who were stationed on the island of
Malta in the Mediterranean, although there were almost no
signs of the disease among the native population. But this
does not prove that Anglo-Saxons are genetically less resistant to polio than Mediterranean peoples. A much more likely
explanation is that the polio virus is widely spread among the
Maltese and that they have all developed immunity at a very
early age, whereas the average Englishman, born into an environment with better sanitation, had not met the virus before.

Similarly, at first sight it appears that American Indians
and Negroes are less resistant to, and react differently to, the
tuberculosis organism than the white races, and that this
might be a genetic difference. It is equally likely, however,
that the white races have been in contact with this tuberculosis menace for thousands of years and that natural selection
has had time to weed out the less resistant, while for the
Negro and the American Indian this process is still at an
early stage. But no conclusion can be reached on this matter
because any study of the problem is bedevilled by the social
and environmental differences between the living conditions
of the majority of people in the racial groups involved.

There is, however, a definitely established genetic factor
involved in natural resistance to malaria, and this is one of
the fascinating features of malarial immunity which make it
worth a special section on its own in a later chapter. But
while this factor is most obvious, naturally, among African
Negroes there is no proof that it is necessarily confined ra-
cially to them.

Still, there are many diseases of pet animals, farm animals, and wild animals which are either rare or unknown
among men, and therefore presumably we have some genetic
resistance to them.

This subchapter on our general and non-specific defences

against invasion, which I feel is like the sort of military operation where a general straightens out his lines or eliminates
an enemy salient before launching a general attack, might
have been written ten days earlier if my wife had not insisted
that the roses must be pruned. My hands on the typewriter
bear witness to the operation, and raise the question, Why
have the many small breaches in my skin caused by the rose
thorns (breaches which are all healing nicely, thank you)
why have they not allowed as many invasions by germs? Obviously there is another defence mechanism at work. Some of
the defence may, of course, be the recognition of organisms
which have entered through the wounds as not-self and their
subsequent elimination. But it is known that this is not the
whole story because it has been proved, by those who do research on wounds and inflammation, that there is a great
deal of activity in the first five minutes after wounding,
whereas a full-scale specific immune reaction may take at
least three to five days to mount.

A superficial wound immediately lays bare two different
systems, the blood system and the lymphoid system, and
both these systems discharge liquid into the wound area. It
was at one time thought that this discharge of liquid was
itself a defence mechanism, a washing away of invading organisms. This is doubted nowadays if only because the liquid
pressure in the lymph system is null and its exposure therefore seems to offer an ideal channel for invasion by organisms
which enter through the wound. The whole mechanism of reaction to a wound and the phenomenon of inflammation has
given rise to enormous research and equally formidable literature describing it. Here and now there is no need to say
more than that quantities of powerful chemicals of many
kinds are rapidly brought to the site of a wound, and kill
many invading organisms on the spot. Most of these chemicals come in the blood stream, which in any case contains
enzymes, primarily circulating for the body's own use and

control, which are quite capable of killing bacteria on the side. There is the organisation of the bodies called platelets, a normal feature of the blood stream, which have been well described as "mobile first-aid boxes"; their arrival is followed by the release of the powerful histamines, which not only kill invaders but also damage the body's own cells. And there are several other mechanisms of lesser importance, too.

Even if an invading organism gets beyond the outer defences and enters the blood or lymph systems, there are general and well-organised systems for dealing with it before the specific immune system need come into play. But these systems differ importantly from what has been mentioned before in that they are systems in which whole cells play the crucial role—these are *cellular* defence systems rather than the "humoral" systems of various chemicals in the blood stream.

The cells involved in these systems are "white" cells, the leucocytes, so called to distinguish them from the "red" cells also seen in the blood under the microscope. But there are many different sorts of white cell, and one of the great difficulties for a layman (meaning simply anyone who is not a physiologist or doctor, and including such people as physicists, chemists, and mathematicians) trying to understand a medical textbook is that the same sort of white cell may be called by several different names at different times for no apparent reason. Thus one type of cell involved in this defence process can be known as a polymorphonuclear leucocyte, a leucocyte, a polymorph, a microphage, a phagocyte, or even a pyrinophil (the last meaning simply that it is a cell which can be stained with a chemical so that it will show up on the microscope slide). This type of cell must not be confused with a mononuclear leucocyte, which is a macrophage, but which, if the writer is careless, likewise gets called a phagocyte and a leucocyte.

For our purpose there are simply two kinds of white cells

which are involved in this non-specific defence system, and they are called phagocytes because they eat things. Their main job in life is to act as the sweepers and cleaners and general garbagemen of the body; they remove cells or bits of cells when they have died; they carry away any bits of small chemicals that get into the blood stream. And that means, of course, that they will ingest invading organisms and disintegrate them before carrying them off to be excreted. They are exceptionally efficient at all this: for instance, where a single pneumococcus germ injected into the abdomen of a mouse will cause a disease which will kill the mouse, 100,000 similar germs injected directly into the blood stream will be cleared away by the phagocytes in a matter of minutes.

This clearing action can be a general one, that is to say, operating on any particles in the blood stream; but it can also be part of the self-recognition mechanism. In this case the action of antibodies on the invading cells, and especially on the surface of the invading cells, renders them more easily taken up and removed by the phagocytes—but that is part of the later story of this book.

The most interesting thing about the phagocytes is that they ingest invading cells, particles, or cell debris in just the same way as an amoeba or protozoa, the simplest of single-celled life forms, gets its food. Indeed, before modern genetics showed that our own phagocytes shared our own genes and nucleic acid structures, it was even suggested that they might be essentially free-living forms that had evolved into a pattern of life in which they lived in other animals' bodies performing their useful scavenging function. But just as an amoeba does not necessarily win the battle when it meets a bacterium, like itself a single-celled creature, so the phagocyte can ingest an invading organism without destroying it. Then the invader shelters and multiplies inside the phagocyte; indeed, the phagocyte actually seems to provide protection against drugs like antibiotics which cannot penetrate the phagocyte's cell wall to act on the bacterium. The tuberculosis germ, mycobacterium tuberculosis, the germs of the brucella family, and many of the most dangerous types of staphylococcus all have this ability to live inside the phagocyte. And viruses and disease-causing organisms like rickettsiae (halfway between viruses and bacteria) have to get inside a living cell in order to "live" and multiply at all.

Considering the general defences of the body against viruses brings us to two further mysteries: "interferon" and fever. Interferon is a substance produced by cells subject to attack by virus; it is treated more fully in a later chapter because it has a fascinating story in its own right. Fever is apparently one of the body's normal reactions to attack by so many different organisms that at first sight it seems reasonable to suppose that it must be a defence mechanism. But many attempts by research workers to show either that germs are less efficient at higher temperatures, or that the other defence mechanisms of the body are made more effective when the temperature is raised, have nearly all proved inconclusive. Deliberately raising the body temperature, producing an artificial fever, certainly seems an effective treatment in some cases of venereal infection, where normally the germs do not produce fever. But the usual practice of reducing the fever in a patient by self-medication or simple medical treatment seems, by and large, to do little harm. There is some evidence that mycobacteria, such as leprosy, concentrate their attacks on the cooler, outer parts of the body, but the true role of fever, if any, remains obscure.

Halfway between the general defences of the body and the specific responses of the immune system is the substance called complement, yet another protein which circulates in the blood. Complement seems to consist of nine distinct pieces, or blocks, which are found in various combinations. In certain circumstances, complement attacks bacteria and other cells by actually making a hole in the cell wall which allows the contents to come out and the cell to be killed. Certainly in some cases the presence of antibody is necessary for this to occur; but at other times, or perhaps with other types of cells, complement may be able to do this alone. There are suggestions that complement may have been, in evolutionary terms, the original mechanism for dealing with invading cells. Other researchers hold that complement has primarily a function in our own control systems and is only secondarily used to help the immune defences when occasion arises.

At the end of this brief outline of the working of the very effective mechanisms which have prevented the rose thorn scratches on my hands from becoming infected, we find no answer to why I can catch measles or tuberculosis when I am quite free of wounds and from simple contact with someone carrying those diseases. Still less is there any explanation as to why, having once caught measles, I should be immune to further attacks from that particular germ. This is the specific immunity which we now believe is conferred by the mechanism that recognises self and not-self. So back to the science of self.

Chapter 3

The Mechanism of the Immune System

All vertebrates, including even the most primitive, have two operationally distinct ways of responding to the introduction of foreign molecules by routes other than into the digestive system. Molecules that evoke responses of these kinds must generally be above a certain size—that is, macromolecules— and they are termed collectively antigens. The two responses that they evoke involve the production of entities with the capacity to react specifically with the antigen causing them. The first of these entities are *lymphocytes*, cells that are normally present in the blood and in lymphoid tissues and of which an average human being contains about a million million. The second are *antibodies*, which are proteins secreted into the blood and the tissue fluids by specialised cells derived from lymphocytes. Antibodies constitute the fraction of blood plasma proteins defined as gamma-globulin, and proteins of this kind have come to be termed immunoglobulins.

This severe, careful definition of the immune response introduces a number of specialised terms and concepts clearly and precisely. It is a definition on which I shall rely because it comes once again from the distinguished immunologist Dr. J. D. Humphrey, and is produced in the 1969 *Annual Report* of the Medical Research Council of Great Britain (see p. 60 of this Report).

The first important point made here is that there are two different ways of reacting to an invasion by foreign bodies. One is at the molecular level, by the production of chemical molecules called antibodies, and the vital point is that a different antibody has to be produced for each different invading organism or particle. In precise terms, the antibody is specific to the antigen.

The second, higher response is at the cellular level. When an antigen is introduced into the body the result is the production of new cells in very large numbers. These cells are likewise specific to the antigen and in ordinary cases of infection are eventually responsible for the production of the large quantities of antibody that may be necessary. Furthermore, after the antibody has disappeared from the body when the attack is over, some of these cells remain in the circulation and in some way provide immunity against a second attack by the same invader. Somehow they carry the "memory" of the shape of the antigen of an invader and can thus reactivate the correct antibody defence very quickly.

There is, however, another important immune mechanism at the cellular level. It is known as "cell-mediated immunity" and it is believed to be the chief mechanism in tissue graft rejection and in some allergies. It involves exactly the same type of cells, but in this reaction the whole cell seems to be involved instead of merely the production of antibody by the cell. This cell-mediated immunity provokes the greatest excitement among, and poses the most difficult questions to, the immunologists at the moment.

The cells involved in all these mechanisms are lymphocytes. They are white cells, very small and apparently simple. They consist, in fact, of hardly more than the nucleus, which contains the genes, and the nucleic acids. Around

this, very little of the other machinery of the cell is visible—
just a small amount of the rich chemical jelly called cytoplasm, and then the cell wall. These are the "small lymphocytes"; they form the majority of the population of a million
million described in Dr. Humphrey's definition. There are,
however, some cells called "large lymphocytes," and their
function is very much the subject of research which is going
on at the moment—which is, I suppose, a polite way of saying that no one is really very sure what they do or how they
do it. In fact, until very recently the function of the small
lymphocytes was unknown; they had been a standing scien-
tific/medical mystery for many years. It had been suggested
that they were involved in the immune processes but there
was no clear confirmation of this until Gowans within the
last ten years performed his experiments of draining off most
of the lymphocytes (more details of these experiments follow later).

The lymphocytes get their name because they are mostly
found in the lymphoid tissues (-cytes is the generic suffix for
words meaning "cells"). Everyone knows what the blood system is, but it is probably worth explaining that the lymphoid
system is equally extensive in the body, although its vessels
are much smaller and its contents are not pumped round
under pressure. The lymphoid system is more like a drainage
system than a supply system: all the peripheral areas of the
body are "drained" by minute channels containing a colorless
liquid, the lymph. The little channels come together in
lymph nodes, very small glands which quite often become
enlarged when there is an infection. Indeed, enlarged lymph
nodes at certain places—behind the ear or under the jaw—
are classical symptoms of certain common infections like
German measles and mumps. The lymphoid system contains
largish organs such as the thymus and the spleen, and it does
eventually connect with the blood stream. But the use of the

term "organs" is perhaps slightly misleading, for it might be more correct to describe the thymus, the spleen, and the mysterious Peyer's patches at the lower end of the intestine as concentrations of lymphoid tissue rather than organs in the sense of the liver or kidneys. The function of these lymphoid tissues is by no means fully explained or understood but there is considerable knowledge now of the operations of the thymus at least.

Antigen and Antibody

The basic method used by the body to combat invasion by some other organism is the production of antibody which is specifically designed against the invader. We have described the invader as "antigen," and we also use the same word to describe those features of the invader's surface or outside structure which enable it to be recognized as an invader, that is to say, as something which is not-self. Because we use this word, and perhaps because there is some emotional connotation about the sound "anti," we tend to think of antigen as a clearly marked flag, rather like the colors of a man-of-war, something which can be "nailed to the mast." In fact, the antigen is simply the shape of the large molecules which make up the surface covering of the invader.

In the basic definition of immune systems at the beginning of this chapter it was stated that immune reactions were only evoked by molecules above a certain size—macromolecules or very large molecules. The point here is that all living organisms are made up of macromolecules; there can be very large molecules which are not part of living matter, but there is no living matter which is not made of very large molecules. The contrast, as far as the immune system is concerned, is that if you inject inorganic molecules into the body—finely ground talcum powder or carbon black—then these large but simply shaped molecules are carried off by the phagocytes and excreted. But the very large molecules that make up living matter usually consist of long chains of subunits with several small side chains attached, and are wound together in a highly complicated three-dimensional shape. This shape shows clefts or bumps, which very often appear to present the most active portions of the molecule to the outside world in some special way so that it can most easily combine with some other equally complicated substance. Similarly, amongst all this folding and bending there may be places where the electric charge appears to be concentrated, making it particularly attractive to another molecule which has an opposite electric potential at some point. Very little of this complicated business has been worked out in any detail. It is still hailed as a triumph when the full structure of an enzyme is described. These full descriptions of macromolecules are more than just a chemical analysis, a listing and numbering of every atom and subunit in the molecule. They give the shape of the molecule in three dimensions and thus enable scientists to gain a much clearer understanding, a visual grasp, of how the thing works. So far only about half a dozen enzymes and a few other important macromolecules such as haemoglobin have been fully described, so our real knowledge of the shape of the molecular world is extremely limited.

But we can at least appreciate that living matter consisting of these macromolecules is a very "shapely" thing when viewed at the molecular level. And it is comparatively easy to visualise how the shape of an invading organism can be distinctive enough for it to be recognised. Likewise we can visualise that an antibody, which is itself a macromolecule, can be constructed so that it is shaped to combine easily with the invader: the antibody will have a lump to fit into a cleft in the invader, or it may have a negatively charged hollow to fit over the positively charged lump on the invader.

It must be emphasised here, in discussing "living" matter and invaders, that antibody can be formed against any macromolecule. This means that it is possible to form antibody not only against an invading organism but also against parts of such an organism, against poisons produced by it (for example, the toxin produced by diphtheria bacilli), or against single "organic" chemicals prepared in the laboratory, as long as they are large enough. (The last is important to the research worker trying to sort out the infinitely complicated mechanisms of the millions of cells and antibodies found in a living animal.)

Because it must have some shape, every cell and every important chemical in all living bodies can be antigen. Although a bacterium appears to be antigen to my body, cells or enzymes from my body appear to be antigen to a fish, or to my dog, or to you. It is more difficult to visualise how the surface of one of my liver cells differs in shape from one of yours, simply because the nucleic acids inside my cells are arranged only slightly differently from those inside yours. But as I should almost certainly reject a graft of your liver there must be some appreciable difference, some external expression of the genetic differences between us. Amid the enormous complexity which we now know to be typical of macromolecules and their convoluted shapes, it is not impossible to imagine subtle differences of arrangement or profile.

The body reacts to the appearance of a foreign macromolecule (or combination of macromolecules as an organism) by making an antibody shaped and charged electrically in such a way that it will physically attach itself to the antigen of the invader. This binding of antibody to antigen, a physical binding together, is the principal way in which the body neutralizes invaders. It has four chief objectives.

1. Antibody agglutinates antigen. This means that antibody pulls together numbers of the invading organisms into clumps so that they cannot spread around the body and multiply. Antibody can do this because it is manufactured in a chain-like form with at least two "combining sites" on each chain and sometimes as many as ten of these combining sites linked together. The combining sites are the places shaped to fit onto a particular feature of the antigen.

2. In many reactions, where the invader is a bacterium of the type called "gram-negative," the binding of antibody onto invader enables one of the other components of the blood, the nine-piece substance known as complement, to punch a hole in the cell wall of the invader and thus destroy it. (This process is termed "lysis.")

3. By combining with the antigen, the antibody makes it easier for the phagocytes to ingest the invaders. It is not known how this is achieved, but it is assumed that the surface of the invader is made either "stickier" or "smoother" to the phagocyte. It is clear that the process of phagocytosis (eating) is speeded up in the presence of antibody, and still more speed is added by the presence of the first four pieces of complement.

4. In dealing with invaders which are not cellular, such as viruses, toxins (poisons), or enzymes produced by invaders, the binding antibody appears literally to neutralize them or destroy their activity by physically covering active sites. Thus it is believed that some viruses use the "spikes" which stick out around them to penetrate the walls of body cells they are trying to invade; in certain electron microscope pictures it is clear that antibody binds onto these spikes, and thus presumably prevents them from penetrating cell walls.

These are the modes of action of antibodies. In principle, a specific antibody is made for each particular type of invader; in practice, however, it is not quite so simple because it is possible to get "cross-reactions." One reason for this is that an invading organism may well have more than one "antigenic determinant." Obviously, the cell walls of different types of bacteria are broadly similar. A bump or hollow on one wall will be very like, may indeed be identical to, a bump or hollow on another. Hence antibody to one bacteria may bind to another kind of bacteria, though the fit at the binding site may be far from perfect. Similarly, two different kinds of antibody can well bind to one and the same invader. The immunologists have concepts of "affinity" and "avidity" for describing in quantitative terms the binding speeds, frequencies, and efficiencies of antibodies and antigens. These terms are widely used in discussing and interpreting their experimental results, but such complications need not disturb the basic concepts.

Antibodies have long been known to exist. In the early days of immunology, when the science was mostly concerned with preparing vaccines against infectious diseases, they could be demonstrated and even, in some sense, seen, by mixing immune blood serum (the treated blood of a person or animal known to have had a disease) with the organisms that caused the disease; then the clumps of bacteria agglutinated together by the antibody would precipitate out of the mixture as visible particles.

Blood is a complex fluid: it contains not only red and white cells, the oxygen-carrying haemoglobin, and all the hormones and enzymes that must be carried round the body for innumerable purposes, but also the antibodies. Many years ago a number of blood components called globulins were identified. The globulins were later split up into three types: alpha, beta, and gammaglobulins, according to the different speeds at which they traveled across a piece of paper when an electric potential was applied. But only in 1939 was it shown that antibody activity resided in the gammaglobulins. From this historical confusion there has arisen a confusion of names. Antibody and gammaglobulin both refer to the same substances; whence they are nowadays called immunoglobulins.

At least five types of immunoglobulin have definitely been discovered, and there is speculation that a sixth may also exist. The normal immunoglobulin, the commonest and lightest in weight, the one to which we usually refer when we speak of antibody, is IgG. IgG simply means immunoglobulin G. Immunoglobulin A, IgA, is rather heavier than IgG; it is the immunoglobulin that is secreted from the body, dealing with cold and influenza germs in the mucus of the nose and respiratory tracts. It is also passed on by all mammalian mothers to their infants in those special first breast feeds containing colostrum.

It is tempting to consider IgM, the biggest and heaviest of the immunoglobulins, simply as five IgG molecules stuck together. This is certainly what it looks like in electron microscope pictures, but the latest chemical work shows that although it does consist chiefly of five large bodies stuck together, there are nevertheless clear differences between the components of IgM and the IgG molecules. IgM is distinguished as being the first antibody to be produced against an invader; its role seems to be that of the shock troops of the defence or, to use a perhaps more accurate analogy, the leader of the counter-attack. Later on, IgG takes over from IgM in becoming the most common antibody against any specific antigen threat.

IgE is the immunoglobulin whose role has been identified most recently. It is the antibody that operates in cases of allergy. IgD is a bit of a mystery. It can clearly be found and distinguished from the other immunoglobulins, but it is never found in large quantities and no one knows what it does. There are rumours and hints about there also being an IgX, but no evidence for its existence has so far been published.

If you read about immunoglobulins in a modern textbook

you will be struck by the continuous use of the term "hetero-geneous." This implies that just about every possible varia-tion has been observed and that there are exceptions to every rule. But it is reasonable that variation should be the chief feature of antibody, as the job of antibody is to be ready to meet any variety of invader. Incidentally, antibodies can themselves be seen as antigens and it is possible to prepare anti-immunoglobulin antibody, which is specific for the class of antibody, say anti-IgM, but not specific for the antibody binding site.

The immunoglobulin IgG is nowadays visualized as con-sisting essentially of two identical parts linked together, each part containing one of the antibody sites where the actual combination with the antigen takes place. Each of the two equal parts contains one string of subunits known as a "heavy chain" and one string known as a "light chain." The heavy chain runs the whole length of both sections, and is also re-sponsible for the formation of the shape of the antibody site. The light chain runs only part of the length of each section. It is not precisely known whether the light chain takes any part in the formation of the antibody site, but the links be-tween the two parts—called sulphide bonds because they are essentially chemical bonds between corresponding sulphur atoms on the two chains—are links between the light chains.

Antibody was originally only visualised like this, because until very recently it was not seen in sufficient detail for any-one to know exactly what it looks like. The steps that led to this conception are a fascinating example of how the immu-nologists go about their work. By using a highly active en-zyme called papain, it was found that IgG from both rabbits and human beings could be split into three equal parts. The three fragments were then separated by the technique of chromatograph, in which a complex mixture is allowed to percolate from the top edge of an absorbent medium, such as paper, to the bottom; the different speeds at which the vari-

IMMUNOGLOBULIN Ig G

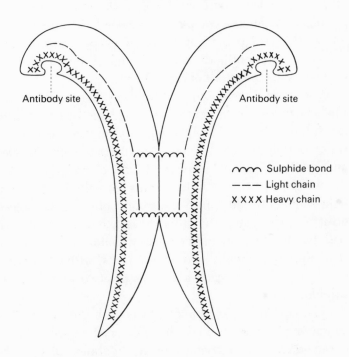

ous components of the mixture travel through the medium enables them to be separated.

Two of these three fragments were discovered to be virtually identical, and each was shown to contain one antibody site by making them combine with the organism against which the original IgG had been prepared. The third fragment had no antibody activity, and furthermore could be made to crystallise. But when the two different fragments were injected into rabbits, it was shown that the rabbits made two different types of antibody—in other words, the two different fragments when regarded as antigens are different again.

If, however, the IgG is treated first with a different enzyme, pepsin (a digestive enzyme found in the stomach), the third fragment, which crystallised in the previous set of experiments, is almost completely digested. Treatment of the remainder with papain again provides two portions, each containing one antibody site and slightly heavier than the fragments in the first set of experiments.

A different technique of splitting big molecules into smaller pieces uses a gentler chemical method that attacks just sulphide bonds. The IgG made by rabbits, treated in this way, splits into two different sets of fragments, one heavy and one light—hence, heavy and light chains. Furthermore, the weight of two heavy fragments plus the weight of two light fragments adds up to the weight of one IgG molecule. So it was suggested that there was a four-chain structure, with two light chains and two heavy chains, pairing off into a structure of essentially two similar parts, with one light and one heavy chain in each and with the two parts joined by sulphide bridges.

The next step was to inject goats with the two antibody-containing fragments and the one crystallisable fragment obtained from the enzyme-splitting treatment of IgG. As in the case of rabbits, the goats developed two sets of antibodies, which in practice means two different antisera.[1] When the same type of IgG was split into heavy and light fragments and these were reacted with the two different types of antiserum, the heavy chains combined with both sorts of antiserum; but the light chains combined only with the antiserum against the antibody-containing fragments. Thus there was no light chain in that fragment from the enzyme-splitting process which could be crystallised.

Further experiments of a similar nature have shown that both IgA and IgM have the heavy and light chain structure, and that the heavy chain is responsible for shaping the antibody site. The role of the light chain appears to be that of stretching out the heavy chain into its most useful shape and keeping it soluble in the blood by preventing it from "curling up" on itself and crystallising.

Probably the most important techniques to be invented by immunology have been the techniques for demonstrating the existence of antibody and then for determining the existence of specific antibody. The basic technique for demonstrating the existence of antibody is also that for rendering animals and people immune to infectious diseases. I have emphasised this already, but it is worth repeating that the scientific demonstration of antibody, or something which operates in the way we believe antibody to operate, is also the extremely useful technique of rendering ourselves immune to dangerous diseases. But as a technique it is clumsy and expensive for laboratory purposes. To the research man a laboratory method of demonstrating antibody was important. And several have been discovered, all utilizing various properties of different sorts of antibody.

In outlining the modes of action of antibodies, one of their chief functions was described as "clumping together" invasive organisms. We guess that this action has some real value in protecting the host from invasion, perhaps in reducing the mobility of the invaders as well as in presenting them to attack by macrophages. This function of clumping—technically agglutination—also provides a way of observing the presence of antibody in the laboratory. If serum containing specific antibody is added to a suspension of bacteria in liquid, the formation of clumps of cells drawn together by the antibody can be observed. Sometimes it can actually be seen by the naked eye, though normally a scientist will use a microscope or hand lens to observe the action. Agglutination is one of the classical techniques of the immunologist.

Agglutination only occurs with whole cells. It can therefore only be used in the study of bacterial diseases and other ailments caused by cellular organisms such as yeasts and fungi. But from diseases it can also be extended to provide techniques for the study of body cells, notably blood cells. Agglutination of red cells by antibody has become, in fact, the standard method of testing and research into blood groups. If we inject the red cells of one person into an animal such as a rabbit or guinea-pig, the animal will develop antibody against the particular type of red cells provided by the donor, A, B, or O, and so on. The antisera taken from the guinea-pig can be used to discover whether samples of blood taken from other human beings are of the same blood group or not. This technique is the basis of blood-grouping for clinical purposes—defining the blood of volunteer donors and matching with accident victims, hospital patients, etc.

By even further extension of the techniques of agglutination, immunology has helped in other fields of science. Forensic science, detective work, has benefited greatly, because it is by these antibody agglutination techniques that the police scientist can tell whether bloodstains on clothing are caused by animal or human blood. Indeed, it is even possible to establish evolutionary relationships between different types of animal by agglutination tests, since antibody against the red blood cells of one species will cause more agglutination among the blood cells of a closely related species and less among cells from a distantly related species.

It is also possible for the immunologist to introduce quantitative measurements of antibody and antigen into his agglutination tests. He prepares a row of test tubes in which he places different quantities of antigen, probably by taking a culture of bacteria and steadily diluting the suspension of organisms in the nutrient liquid, so that the first test tube contains a dilution of 1 in 10, the second 1 in 20, the third 1 in 40, and so on. He then puts exactly equal amounts of serum in each tube from a pipette. The last tube in the series to show agglutination just visible to the naked eye is taken as the reference point—the amount that will be taken to contain one "unit" of antibody or antigen. The whole process can be carried out the other way round, with different dilutions of serum or steadily decreasing concentrations of antibody, and equal drops of bacterial culture or equal amounts of antigen.

One of the surprising by-products of all the research into influenza virus in the 1930's and 1940's was the discovery that this virus had the power of agglutinating red blood cells in a very similar way to the action of antibody in clumping cells. This not only gave a method for testing for the presence of influenza virus and then quantifying the amounts of virus present. It also made possible the demonstration of the presence of antibody to influenza virus, for the antibody binds itself to the virus particles and then the virus can no longer agglutinate red cells. In this case, by an odd reversal, it is the prevention of "haemagglutination"—the clumping of red blood cells—that can be used to test for the presence and quantity of antibody. It has since been shown that other viruses of the same family as influenza virus, myxovirus, have the power of haemagglutination. Consequently, these techniques can be used also in research into the mumps virus and the virus that causes Newcastle disease in chickens. (Nowadays we must add many of the pox and arbor viruses to the list of viruses capable of causing haemagglutination.)

It was obvious from the early days of immunology that a simple test for the presence of antibody might be to cultivate a bacterium in a laboratory glass dish containing a layer of nutrient substance on which the bacteria could feed. Placing drops of a serum which was expected to contain antibody specific against the bacteria on this dish, small patches of the bacteria ought to be killed by the antibody and this should be visible. This procedure is, in fact, quite practicable. The areas of killed bacteria show up as "plaques," little circles of a colour different from the rest of the plate, indicating where the bacteria have been killed. The problem, however, is that there is nothing in the process to prove that it is the antibody in the serum which has killed the bacteria. It may be some other substance as yet unknown to science. The point is proved by the famous story of Fleming's discovery of penicillin when he spotted that such plaques had been formed on laboratory cultures of bacteria, though in his case it was an accidental, external organism which had caused the change. However, the basic piece of equipment for this type of study —the glass dish containing a layer of nutrient material, usually the sugary jelly agar—has developed into what is probably the immunologist's most important single item of technique.

In cases where the antigen is not part of a whole cell, that is to say, when the antigen is a virus or one of the large biomolecules like a protein, the binding of antibody to antigen produces small solid particles which come out of solution in the serum. These are visible to the naked eye, at least *en masse,* although each individual particle of antigen-antibody may be only just visible to the electron microscope. The combination of antibody and antigen "precipitates," just as a chemical reaction between two elements often forms a visible precipitate. So, if the immunologist fills the bottom of a test tube with antiserum, and then carefully layers on top of this a solution containing the antigen, a white disc of "precipitate" will appear where the two mixtures meet. There will be a visible white band in the test tube and he will have demonstrated that antibody specific to that particular antigen was present. A slightly more sophisticated version of this test is to put the antiserum in agar jelly or to place a column of agar above the antiserum in the bottom of the tube. Then, when he puts the antigen solution into the top of the tube the precipitate (also known as the precipitin band) will form in the agar at the point where antibody and antigen meet as they diffuse in opposite directions through the agar. But in this sort of experiment the diffusion of antibody and antigen and their mutual interaction and precipitation is only observed in one direction; only one conclusion can be drawn, namely, that antibody specific to that antigen is present.

By observing diffusion and precipitation in two dimensions, much more interesting results can be obtained. To achieve this the immunologist takes the traditional laboratory glass dish and covers the base with a thin layer of agar. He then makes three little "wells" or circular holes in the agar. In one well he places a drop of antiserum, in another antigen. Antibody and antigen diffuse out from the wells into the agar and at some point they meet, combine, and form a precipitate. Again, the precipitate can be seen with the naked eye, white in the darkish agar. In fact, since the antibody and antigen have diffused out of their wells equally in all directions, they meet and form their white precipitate all along a line approximately halfway between the two wells. This proves that antibody specific to the antigen was present.

But so far we have ignored the existence of the third well. If at the start of the experiment the immunologist had placed an unknown antigen in the third well, a number of interesting possibilities begin to emerge. If, for instance, just one continuous white line of precipitate appears—it will be a curved line rather similar to a segment of a circle centered on the well containing the antiserum—then the antigen in the third well is identical with the antigen in the second well, because both have reacted identically with the highly specific antibody in the antiserum.

It may well happen that one continuous line is formed, but also "branches" or "spurs" of white precipitate may appear, apparently growing out of the main line. This shows that although the two test wells contain identical antigen, which reacts with a component of the antiserum along a continuous line, there must, too, be some other component present which cross-reacts with the antibody, or which reacts with some other antibody in the antiserum.

Here we have a testing technique which is not only valuable to the immunologist but can also be used by other branches of science for purposes of detecting, with extreme accuracy, the presence or absence of biological materials. A simple example is its application in deciding whether a patient has a particular infectious disease, say smallpox. A quantity of smallpox virus would be put into one well; smallpox antiserum (serum containing anti-smallpox antibody) would be put into another well; while material from the blood of the person suspected of having caught smallpox would be put into the third well. If a continuous line of precipitate is formed, there is smallpox virus in the material from the suspect. The actual practice in clinical cases, where the health authorities are coping with an outbreak of smallpox, is more sophisticated than this; but the principle is the same and the technique allows cases of smallpox or other infectious diseases to be identified with certainty long before clinical symptoms have appeared.

However, materials from living bodies are normally very complex, containing many different substances. The diffusion technique has to be made more sophisticated to cope with most research problems. Immuno-electrophoresis is an example of such a highly sophisticated technique. Instead of the traditional round glass dish, a rectangular dish is used with a layer of agar on the bottom. A small well is made in the agar towards one end. An electric potential is then applied across the agar. The various components of the serum diffuse along the dish at different speeds according to the slightly different electric potentials possessed by the different kinds of molecules. Thus the serum becomes spread out with each different component in a slightly different position along the dish.

Next, the immunologist cuts a trench in the agar along the length of the dish. Into this trench he runs, perhaps, anti-serum prepared in a rabbit against all the human serum he has placed in the original well. The different components of the serum will react with the many different antibodies in the antiserum and a whole sequence of arching white lines of precipitate will be formed at many different places along the length of the dish.

This technique, again, has been used for many research projects which are outside the scope of immunology. It has been shown, for example, that normal human blood serum contains more than thirty different substances which are antigenically distinct. It clearly shows up the different types of globulin—alpha, beta, and gamma—and it distinguishes between the different types of gammaglobulin, distinct lines being formed by IgA, IgG, and IgM.

The immunoglobulins are proteins, which means that they are examples of a very common class of molecules in living bodies. Proteins are long molecules made up of strings of subunits called amino acids, and there are only twenty different amino acids. The stringing together of amino acids to make proteins is the chief "manufacturing" job of the living cell. The operation is carried out under the "instructions" of the nucleic acids in the chromosomes, the order of amino acids being decided by the order of the subunits in the nucleic acids. The actual process of joining up the amino acids is carried out by small particles called ribosomes, which are often linked together on the messenger RNA to make poly-ribosomes.

There is no doubt that antibody is made primarily in the

plasma cells, which are found particularly in the lymphoid tissues, such as spleen, bone marrow, and the lymph nodes. Obviously these plasma cells, situated chiefly in the medulla region of the lymph nodes, are specially adapted for the production of large amounts of protein. The manufacturing area, the cytoplasm, is unusually large. It is full of the membranes known as endoplasmic reticulum, and under the electron microscope very large numbers of ribosomes and polyribosomes can be seen. The whole cell is in fact specially formed for a rapid, large-scale protein production. By taking antibody IgG from one animal and injecting it into another, it can be proved that the protein it manufactures is antibody. The second animal naturally manufactures antibody against the foreign protein in the shape of an antiserum to the first animal's antibody. The second antibody can be stained with a substance (fluorescein) that will fluoresce brilliantly when subjected to ultraviolet light. The stained antiserum is then applied to the tissues of the original animal and the original antibody of course immediately combines with it. Therefore, under a fluorescent microscope, wherever a glow is seen the antiserum from the second animal is combining with the antibody of the first animal. In this way it can be shown clearly where the first animal has most antibody (in the lymphoid tissues, and particularly in the cytoplasm of plasma cells in the lymph nodes). Indeed, it can even be shown by this method that these plasma cells are producing antibody more actively if the animal has recently been stimulated by an attack from another antigen.

But where do the plasma cells come from? And how do they know what antibody to make at any particular time? Currently these are the crucial questions. At present the most favoured answer to the first is that plasma cells develop from lymphocytes, which also generate the essential information as to which antibody to manufacture. The second question, referring to the cellular mechanism, resolves then into a discussion of the lymphocytes.

Lymphocytes

The lymphocytes are the white cells found mainly in the lymphoid tissues, but also in many other parts of the body. They come in various sizes. There are small lymphocytes, large lymphocytes, and lymphocytes that appear to be in-between. But 95 percent of them are small. Since no one knows exactly what function a large lymphocyte performs, and since, indeed, it may be no more than an enlarged version of a small lymphocyte capable of transforming itself back again into the small version, I shall concentrate exclusively on the small one. There are a trillion small lymphocytes in the body normally; yet, only ten years ago no one knew what their function could be.

But in the last ten years the lymphocyte has moved right to the center of the picture so far as the immunologist is concerned. The lymphocyte is *the* "immunologically competent" cell, the cell whose function it is to organise the immune response, the self-defence system. The small lymphocyte carries within itself not only the power to recognise not-self, but also the power to initiate the destruction of not-self. It is, moreover, the small lymphocyte that is the carrier of immunological memory—the readiness to mount a very quick counter-attack against any antigen that has been met before. Finally, the small lymphocyte provides the specificity that characterises the immune response, the ability to react in a different way to every different antigen, each response being specific to the particular antigen invading at the time.

Small lymphocytes derive from stem cells in the bone marrow. From the marrow they move into the circulation of the body. They can be found in the blood and in the lymphatic system, in spleen and lymph nodes particularly, but also in the lungs and most other organs, as well as among the interstices of cells in the limbs. In fact, they circulate round the entire body. They are very small cells consisting of little more than the nucleus (containing the nucleic acids in the shape of chromosomes), surrounded by little of the manufacturing equipment which is a feature of many cells. But there are very large numbers of lymphocytes, and together they make up nearly 1 percent of the total body weight.

It has now been established that there are two separate populations of lymphocytes. One set is comparatively short-lived. These exist as individual cells for only a few days before continuing the line by generating identical daughter cells. The other population consists of cells that are surprisingly long-lived—they may last as individuals for at least ten years, and possibly even twenty. It is mostly these long-lived cells that circulate continuously round the body, reaching the farthest, most peripheral areas via the blood stream, then returning to the lymphatic system and recirculating again.

The two populations differ in yet another way, for the long-lived lymphocytes have all passed through, or been derived from, the thymus. All lymphocytes originate from stem cells in the bone marrow (and also in the liver during foetal life). The stem cell divides into two identical cells. At least one of these daughter cells goes off into the body as a small lymphocyte. It then moves either to the thymus or straight into the lymphatic system, migrating eventually to one of the lymph nodes. There it joins similar cells concentrated in certain areas. The primary job of the lymphocytes that have not passed through the thymus is to develop, when stimulated by antigen, into plasma cells, the producers of antibody.

Those lymphocytes that go to the thymus, or develop in the thymus from stem cells that have taken the same path, multiply rapidly in the thymus (they are often called thymo-cytes). Much of the inside of the thymus (although admit-tedly it is not a very large organ in human adults) consists of little but closely packed lymphocytes, the vast majority of which never leave the thymus; they simply die there, and apparently their material is reused to make more lympho-cytes. However, a small number do leave. These are the long-lived lymphocytes that circulate and recirculate around the body. When they are not circulating they are almost all packed into the lymph nodes and the spleen. In the lymph nodes the thymus-derived lymphocytes concentrate in sepa-rate areas from the short-lived lymphocytes—in fact, in the so-called thymus-dependent areas.

The tasks of the long-lived, or thymus-derived, lympho-cytes are several. It is virtually certain, for one thing, that they carry the immunological memory. It is also these long-lived lymphocytes that have the function of organising the cell-mediated immune reaction, for the rejection of grafts and transplants and for those reactions of "delayed hypersen-sitivity" that include allergies. Exactly how they operate in rejecting grafts is not clear, but a rejected transplant usually shows a massive invasion by the host's lymphocytes, and most of the other evidence points in the same direction.

It is probable, though not finally proved, that within the lymph nodes the thymus-derived lymphocytes (or T-lymphocytes, as some authorities call them) cooperate in some way with the short-lived lymphocytes (sometimes called B-lymphocytes) when antigen comes to stimulate their activity. It seems likely that the long-lived lymphocytes, per-haps in combination with phagocytes, present the antigen in a way that stimulates the short-lived lymphocytes to trans-form themselves, first into large lymphocytes and then into plasma cells that produce the antibody to the particular antigen.

It is certain that the long-lived lymphocytes produce a certain factor upon meeting antigen—the so-called humoral factor—that affects the phagocytes, and particularly the macrophages, by changing their mobility. The result, conceivably, is to concentrate the invading antigen in the lymphatic system and lymph nodes, where it can be met with the full weight of the immune defences. It is also possible that the long-lived lymphocytes produce some substance that affects the general condition of the body around a site of invasion. They may be responsible for increasing the permeability of the walls of the small capillary blood vessels, thus allowing increased movement of defending cells to the area of invasion. It is suggested here that the production of a particular, and only recently recognised, type of gammaglobulin, IgE, may be part of this operation, especially when it is concerned with the kind of inflammation typical of allergy.

All these actions put together really amount to the original statement that the lymphocyte is the immunologically competent cell; it is the lymphocyte which is responsible for the specific defence provided by the body against any particular invader. This leaves wide open such questions as, How does the body recognise an invader? or How can the lymphocytes cope with different kinds of invaders? But before giving some of the immunologists' answers to these problems, let us see how the crucial role of the lymphocyte was discovered.

In the late 1950's no one knew the role of the small lymphocytes in the body. But between 1957 and 1959 Dr. James Gowans at Oxford evolved a technique which at least opened up the possibility of studying their activity. He placed a cannula (a little plastic tube) into the thoracic duct of a number of rats in a way that continually drained the contents of the duct out of each animal. The thoracic duct is one of the chief channels in the lymphatic system, and the drained liquid proved to be small, medium, and large lymphocytes in lymph fluid. The lymph fluid was fed back into the animal, but the cells were separated and kept for study. It became apparent that on the first few days of drainage the rat would produce as many as 100 million lymphocytes each day, and all but 5 percent of these were small lymphocytes. The number of circulating lymphocytes inside the rat notably diminished only after several days; but there was still a huge population of lymphocytes inside the animal, all apparently safely bound to the various tissues in which they reside. Merely a few areas of the lymph nodes—the areas we now call thymus-dependent—were depleted of lymphocytes. If the drainage channel was closed, it would take several weeks for the number of circulating small lymphocytes to get back to normal. On the other hand, if the lymphocytes taken out of the rat were "labelled" with radioactive chemicals, or if radioactively labelled small lymphocytes from another rat of the same strain were injected into a drained rat, it was immediately obvious that these circulating small lymphocytes could pass from blood stream to lymphatic system and back. In fact, it was clear that their main activity was simply to circulate round and round the body, and they had a very long life, certainly as much as ten years. So there were two populations of lymphocytes, one circulating, one sedentary, but still no clue as to what function they performed.

The original vital lead to the role of the lymphocyte had come from the development of Medawar's earlier work on tolerance. His former colleagues Billingham and Brent were examining the system known as "graft-versus-host" reaction—a system in which the graft rejects the host (instead of vice versa) and causes a wasting disease in it. And they noticed that lymphocytes from the graft appeared to be invading the host.

Gowans therefore chose a very pure strain of rats, so inbred that they were all virtually identical twins and could accept grafts from each other; for the moment I shall call them A/A rats. He then crossbred some of them to get A/B rats. These hybrids would accept grafts from A/A rats because to them A antigens were self, but the parents could not accept grafts from the children because they found B foreign. Gowans demonstrated that, firstly, an injection of small lymphocytes, obtained by thoracic-duct drainage from the A/B hybrid rats, would cause "graft-versus-host" disease in the A/A parents, but not vice versa. He then made certain newborn A/A rats tolerant of hybrid tissue (in the way Medawar had done) by injecting them with bone marrow cells from hybrids, and grafted hybrid tissue onto them. Lymphocytes from the thoracic ducts of these tolerant rats did not then cause "graft-versus-host" disease in the hybrid donors of the graft; in other words, it was the lymphocytes that carried the "tolerance," just as it had been lymphocytes that carried "intolerance" and caused "graft-versus-host" disease in the first experiments.

To be doubly sure, Gowans subsequently injected lymphocytes from A/A animals that had not been made tolerant into the tolerant animals carrying grafts from the hybrids—the grafts were rejected. Furthermore, still obtaining his supplies of lymphocytes from thoracic-duct drainage, he showed that this reversal or abolition of tolerance was in no way dependent on the presence of large lymphocytes, but only on the presence of adequate numbers of small lymphocytes.

This, however, only showed that lymphocytes are responsible for "cell-mediated" immune responses—the responses of graft rejection and allergy or hypersensitivity. To prove that the small lymphocytes of the circulating type were also the "memory" cells required an additional series of experiments. They were carried out, with similar results, during the past few years, again led by Gowans using similar meth-

ods. It had seemed dubious, at first, whether the lymphocytes by themselves were responsible for those immune responses requiring the production of antibody, since antibody
activity was only slightly depressed by continuous drainage
of the thoracic duct. But when a set of rats that had not been
drained were given an injection of a bacteriophage (a virus
that infects a common bacteria of the gut), they reacted in
the usual way by a comparatively slow development of antibody which eventually eliminated the invader. Then the
level of the particular antibody in the blood stream slowly
died away. About a year afterwards the rats were challenged
with the same antigen and, in the proper way of an immune
response to a secondary challenge, they rapidly manufactured large quantities of the required antibody and dealt
with the invader. However, some of the rats that had been
"primed" with the antigen had their circulating lymphocytes
drained off through the thoracic duct. These lymphocytes
were injected into a set of rats which had not been primed
with the antigen but had been irradiated with enough X-rays
to destroy all their own lymphocytes. The irradiated rats
were then given the bacteriophage antigen. They reacted by
producing antibody as fast as the donors themselves. The
donors' lymphocytes had proved that they carried the "memory" of the antigen into rats deprived of all their own lymphocytes by irradiation.

Similarly, lymphocytes from rats primed against tetanus
toxoid were injected into mice which had been given enough
radiation to kill them, although they were still capable of
surviving a week or so. The drained lymphocytes had been
incubated very briefly in test tubes with the tetanus toxoid
but were thoroughly washed before being injected into the
mice. After the injection of the rat lymphocytes, and with all
their own lymphocytes destroyed, the mice were given tetanus toxoid, the antigen in this case. Two or three days later,

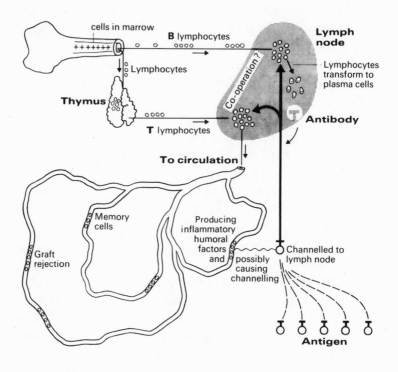

the spleens of the mice were found to be filled with plasma cells which were clearly of *rat* origin and busy making antibody to the tetanus toxoid.

Naturally this is not a full list of all the experiments during the last ten years devoted to establishing that the lymphocyte is the immunologically competent cell. However, these have been the crucial tests that have established the role and behavior of the two populations of lymphocytes.

A further very important development has taken place recently affecting these two populations. Although the work of Robert Good and many others had established the "two-system" nature of the immune mechanism several years ago, there had remained doubt as to whether two entirely different populations of lymphocytes did exist, and in particular the practical problem of deciding to which population any particular lymphocyte belonged was unsolved. Now, however, different antigens have been discovered on the lymphocytes themselves. Thymus-derived lymphocytes have their own type of antigen—the "theta" antigen—and in December 1970 Mitchison and his group announced the discovery of an antigen peculiar to B-lymphocytes, in the mouse at least.

The method by which this problem has been solved itself opens up certain further possibilities. Since the two kinds of lymphocytes have different antigens, it is possible to prepare specific antisera against each population. When one population has been eliminated the activities of the other can be observed in more detail; in particular, it should be possible to discover more about the cooperation between the two populations in immune reactions by observing what does *not* happen when one population has been removed.

A parallel discovery announced in August 1970, comes from one of the best known American immunological teams, the group led by Edward A. Boyse at the Sloan-Kettering Institute for Cancer Research in New York.[2] What they have established is that skin cells (at least in the mouse, but this is unlikely to be confined to one species) have antigens of their own, antigens that are apparently peculiar to skin cells and that are not present on other cells of the same individual if those cells are performing different functions. To be more precise, they have shown that skin cells have different antigens to marrow and lymphoid cells of the same individual.

To demonstrate this, Boyse's group used principles and techniques similar to those used by the Medawar group in establishing the science of self—the technique of producing artificial tolerance and measuring effects by observing the speed of rejection of skin grafts. They have shown, in fact, that animals which have been made tolerant to blood, marrow, and spleen cells from another individual can still reject skin grafts from the same donor individual. Therefore, the skin cells must carry antigens recognisable to the host which are not carried by the cells to which the host has been made tolerant.

The long-term importance of this discovery and its techniques may not lie so much in the field of immunology as in the science of cell biology and the elucidation of the great problem of how cells differentiate in any developing creature. This is one of the basic issues of all modern biology: everything starts as one, then two, and then four identical cells formed from the fusion of a male sperm with a female ovum; the question is how their descendants differentiate into liver cells, brain cells, muscle cells, nerve cells, and so on. Boyse himself, in publishing his discovery, writes: "One important implication of these newly recognised antigenic systems is that they may aid in the understanding of the way in which cells identify one another and so assemble themselves systematically into biological structures." [3] Similarly, the discovery of the theta-antigen on the thymus-derived lymphocyte may help us elucidate the role and action of the thymus, for it is presumably due to the action of the thymus that this exterior manifestation of the inner genetic structure is somehow exposed.

We cannot, realistically, predict what these essentially immunological advances will reveal in the field of cell biology. Probably it will prove a good example of the unpredictability that results from applying the techniques of one scientific discipline in the field of another.

The Reaction to Antigen

Like everything else in immunology (and for that matter in most other sciences), answers to one set of questions simply lead to another even more interesting set. What is the nature of immunological memory? How can the lymphocytes prepare antibody against every possible antigen? What actually happens when antigen meets lymphocyte?

No one knows the quick answers. But the current theories are based on the slogan: "One cell, one antibody." We visualise any single individual lymphocyte as carrying (probably on its surface) just one antibody. Whatever happens to it, whatever antigen it may meet, this type of antibody is the only one it will ever produce; furthermore, all the cells descended from it will produce and carry only this one type of antibody. It therefore follows that only an antigen which fits closely to the antibody on this particular cell will affect its behaviour and cause it to react. The precise reaction of the lymphocyte meeting an antigen fitting its antibody depends, of course, on which type of lymphocyte it is. For instance, it may turn into a plasma cell producing vast quantities of that particular type of antibody only if it is the short-lived type.

An antigen enters the body and in due course meets the lymphocytes. It reacts with those lymphocytes carrying antibody that matches with, or fits, the "antigenic determinants" on the invader. Assuming that this particular antigen has not appeared in the body before, there will only be a small number of lymphocytes carrying antibody which matches the new antigen quite closely, and probably even fewer which fit it exactly. Nevertheless, if the fit is close enough, the lymphocyte is "triggered" into action. No one knows what this triggering mechanism is, but its results are clear enough. The lymphocytes affected by the antigen start proliferating, and as they increase in numbers they take up, and attach themselves to, more and more of the invading antigen. Naturally, only the circulating, long-lived T-lymphocytes meet the antigen, react, and start proliferating.

In a successful immune reaction, that is, one which is successful in clearing the body of the antigen, the role of the circulating lymphocytes is first of all to recognize the invader as not-self and multiply themselves sufficiently; and, in cooperation with the macrophages, probably to activate the short-lived lymphocytes resident in the lymph nodes to transform themselves into plasma cells and start them producing large quantities of the specifically appropriate antibody, which will inactivate all the remaining invading antigen.

In this theory it is, in a real sense, the antigen, the invader, which selects those lymphocytes it will trigger into reaction. This is therefore known as the selective theory of antibody production. It implies one very fundamental fact, namely, that our bodies contain, from the start, a number of lymphocytes carrying antibody to every possible antigen. It also implies that all the production of antibody, and all the immune reactions to any particular antigen, are performed by the direct descendants of those lymphocytes which originally carried the antibody specific to that antigen. The descendants of one particular cell which multiplies by dividing itself are theoretically all identical (that is, unless a mutation takes place by some accident in the reproduction and replication of the nucleic acid). Such identical cells deriving from one original progenitor are called a clone. Clonal reproduction, where all the descendants are identical, is similar to vegetative reproduction commonly practised by gardeners with cuttings. It differs essentially from sexual reproduction, which mixes the genetic material and produces offspring different from the progenitors. Hence this theory of the immune reaction is also called the clonal theory.

The clonal theory derives basically from the work of Neils Jerne, a Danish biologist who, when working at the California Institute of Technology, discovered that horses had a minute amount of antibody against a particular antigen before he had injected them with the antigen. Sir Macfarlane Burnet developed this observation into a full-blown theory. It was taken up by the famous American geneticist Joshua Lederberg, and first given some experimental foundation by Lederberg and "Gus" Nossal, the most brilliant protégé of Sir Macfarlane Burnet, now his successor as director of the Hall Institute in Melbourne, Australia.

It took at least ten years before the clonal theory became widely accepted. Jerne made his observations in 1955. The theory was propounded around 1957. It only gained wide acceptance at the Cold Spring Harbor Symposium in 1967. The previous theory, which it has overcome, was the so-called instructive theory, according to which the antigen in some way impressed its shape on the lymphocytes, or antibody producers, and "instructed" them by this reaction into producing antibody against the specific antigen.

Of course, the immediate question arises, How on earth does the body provide itself with at least some examples of every possible type of antibody it can need before it has even met the antigens? Here the immunologists have their little joke. This remarkable range of antibody is provided, they reply, by GOD. And then they explain that GOD is the acronym for "Generator of Diversity." A group of cells must arise at some stage of development when there is the possibility of exceptionally rapid diversification.

The problem of cellular differentiation—why some of our original undifferentiated cells turn into liver cells performing specific functions, while others turn into muscle, nerve, or brain cells—is one of the great unsolved problems of biology, as I have already stressed. The immunologist adds a complication of his own. He holds that the cells that are going to be

stem cells in the bone marrow must at some time differentiate among themselves into cells that are going to produce
different types of antibody. And since there are so many
types of antibody, this diversification must be very fast.
Somehow or other these cells must be varied at a great rate
or alternatively, if the information needed to make all the
possible antibodies is contained in the DNA (the nucleic
acid of the genes), then different parts of the genes, each
responsible for a different type of antibody, must be
switched on and off in a manner difficult to imagine. It is,
however, typical of the speed and excitement of immunology
that since I started writing this book, an important new development in the argument has been published. It appeared
in the latest edition of the *Atlas of Protein Sequence and
Structure* (1969; edited by Margaret Dayhoff) and is essentially a computer calculation demonstrating the possibility
that the information for all antibodies might be contained in
the DNA of the genes, and that a satisfactory evolutionary
picture could be drawn of the development of antibodies in
the form we now know them.

But to return to the body's reaction to the arrival of antigen: it is reasonably clear that the encounter between antigen and a lymphocyte-bearing antibody that matches it does
not necessarily produce a successful immune reaction. The
triggering of the lymphocyte can be towards tolerance or towards immune reaction. This is the moment of recognition of
self or not-self. No one knows what "triggering" is, and all
one can say is that it must be the local circumstances of the
moment that affect the decision whether "to fight or die" (in
the phrase of a well-known immunologist). If the lymphocyte decides to fight, does it go into the mode of fighting that
we call cell-mediated immunity, the type of defensive reaction that applies to graft rejection and allergy? Or does it go
into the mode of fighting called humoral immunity, the acti-

vation of antibody production in the lymph nodes? Even within the fighting mode of cell-mediated immunity, there seems to be the possibility of variation after triggering— graft rejection apparently involves the "good" development of antibody in the IgG form, whereas allergy or hypersensitivity reactions seem to include the production of antibody in the "bad" IgE form.

That it is literally local circumstances which sometimes decide the result of triggering can be seen from experiments which show that the same antigen when introduced through the nose will result in the production of IgE; when introduced through the buttock or lower gut will lead to the production of antibody in the IgG form.

In auto-immune disease, where the body apparently produces antibody to some of its own components, triggering leads to the "wrong" reaction. So virtually all we can say about triggering at the present stage of research is that the meeting of antigen with antibody on the lymphocyte changes the lymphocyte's reactivity to the antigen.

A normal successful immune reaction, however, can be defined as the triggering of the circulating lymphocyte so that it proliferates and then acts to concentrate the antigen in the lymph nodes where the plasma cells, derived from short-lived lymphocytes, will produce large quantities of the appropriate antibody. It is this concentration of the antigen that is the vital part of a successful immune reaction. Once it has been achieved in the lymph nodes, the presence of the antigen stimulates short-lived lymphocytes to develop into plasma cells; obviously it is physically easier for the antibody to inactivate the invader if the latter has been brought to the antibody production site.

The cooperation of long-lived lymphocytes, short-lived lymphocytes, and macrophages in this concentration and in the process of antibody production is the subject of much of the most advanced current research in immunology. It seems likely that some of the lymphocytes are actually responsible for concentration of antigen by binding it physically to themselves and then bringing it to the receptor sites, the antibody, on the surface of other lymphocytes. Or it may be that lymphocytes "present" antigen to macrophages or antibody in some way that makes the inactivation of the antigen more effective. It is quite possible that electrostatic charges on the various molecules of antibody and antigen, and changes in the charges caused by binding, may be one of the mechanisms involved.

The process which we laymen describe as immunisation and which we practise on ourselves and on our children must now be fitted into this picture. What we call immunisation is technically described as priming. We are interested in preventing our children from "catching" polio, and so we have them immunised. What we do, then, is to expose the body to the polio virus antigen in a safe form. This exposure causes the triggering off of the appropriate specific lymphocytes and the procedure described above as a normal successful immune response. The body, after this first exposure, or priming, is then ready to mount the extremely rapid, overwhelming secondary immune response when it meets the polio antigen for the second or any subsequent time. To stop anyone "catching" polio we have to prime the body so that any meeting with polio in the natural course of events will elicit this rapid and powerful secondary response, eliminating the invading polio virus before it has any chance to establish itself inside the cells and start multiplying.

The priming is necessary because the normal immune response is a comparatively slow process when the body meets an antigen for the first time; it is rapid only when it is a secondary response. The classical experimental exposition of the speed of the primary response is done by injecting red blood cells of sheep into a mouse. The mouse's blood is then tested at regular intervals for the presence of antibody specific against sheep red blood cells—a simple example of the haemagglutination test in which the mouse blood is mixed with more sheep red blood cells in a test tube. This plainly shows that it takes several days for any considerable quantity of the specific antibody to appear in the mouse blood. In human terms, this slowness of the immune reaction may well mean that a person has died from a massive invasion of some disease organism before the immune defences have had time to come fully into operation. Typically in the case of infected wounds, the invading streptococcus has multiplied more rapidly than the defending lymphocytes have proliferated and produced their antibody. Fortunately, however, there are the body's more general non-specific defence methods (described in the preceding section), which can usually hold the invader under at least some sort of control until the immune defence can reach its fully developed state and produce really large quantities of antibody specific against the invader. When the defences hold until the antibody can eliminate the invader, then we have had an attack of whatever disease it is and we have recovered. This leaves a large amount of antibody available. In addition, a large number of cells specifically directed against that particular invader have been produced by proliferation from the original stem cells. Any immediate attempt to reinvade will therefore find the defences in a highly active state. Slowly, however, the antibody level subsides, and even more slowly, as they come to the end of their long lifespan, the number of lymphocytes carrying the specific antibody must decline.

But if at any time during the first few years after an invasion, the same invader once more enters the body, the specific antibody can immediately be manufactured in very large quantities. This is the secondary response to an antigen, and the antibody will appear in large quantities in the blood during the first few hours after the invader has appeared.

Plainly the body carries a "memory" of the antigen and of the appropriate response to it. This memory is carried in the small lymphocytes, as Gowans's experiments showed. The simplest explanation of memory, and the one most favoured by the immunologists at the moment, is that once an invasion has taken place and the lymphocytes carrying the specific antibody have been triggered into reactive proliferation, there will always be a comparatively large number of lymphocytes carrying that antibody in the circulation. An extension of this idea is the theory that the original meeting of antigen and lymphocytes and the process of triggering produces some slight change in the first generation of proliferating lymphocytes and all subsequent cells of that clone, so that the lymphocytes are thereafter primed in some way for immediate action against the antigen. The circulating lymphocytes which stay in the body after the first attack is over are mostly of the primed type and able to mount their counter-attack more speedily.

"Memory" and "priming," whatever they may finally turn out to mean in physico-chemical terms of change in the numbers or in the state of small lymphocytes, are in any case the basis of practical clinical immunisation. The essential feature of immunisation against measles, smallpox, typhoid, or any other disease is, consequently, that the antigen(s) defining the organisms causing the disease should be introduced into the body in some comparatively harmless fashion. After this has been done, the body is ready to mount the extremely rapid and highly effective secondary response if ever those antigens appear again. Such an understanding of the situation can explain many of the apparent anomalies of immunisation, which often puzzle the layman. Thus, it is not necessary to introduce the exact germ which causes a disease in order to provide immunity: in smallpox vaccination it is the "vaccinia" virus which is introduced into the body rather than the actual organism, "variola major," which causes the disease. The antigens on a vaccinia particle are sufficiently like those on an actual smallpox virus to prime the defences into a state capable of producing the secondary response. In another way, it is sufficient to prime the body against the toxin produced by the diphtheria bacillus rather than against the bacillus itself, since it is the toxin that damages the body rather than the bacillus; in any case, the diphtheria bacillus has a rather special defence against antibody in the shape of an unusual coating to its cell walls.

By the same token a virus-like influenza, which has the ability to mutate rather rapidly with time so that mutations produce different antigens on the surface, has a distinct advantage in evolutionary terms, because bodies which are primed against one type of virus have little or no protection when the same essential virus arrives wearing a different type of antigenic shaping on its exterior. It is quite often possible to tell whether a person was born before 1918 by the presence in his blood of residual quantities of antibody against the "Spanish 'flu" virus which swept the world immediately after the First World War. But this antibody will probably offer no protection against the more recent mutant which causes "Asian 'flu." If (or should it be "when"?) the immunologists, probably working with the molecular biologists, finally define the exact shape and chemical nature of antigens at the atomic and molecular levels, it might even be possible to immunise people without using living organisms at all, simply by injecting synthesized antigens.

When the immune reaction is of the cell-mediated type, as in the graft rejection process, very little is known for certain of the mechanisms which follow the meeting of antigen and antibody-carrying lymphocytes. About all that can be said with certainty is that there is production of antibody against the donor cells and that there is invasion of the graft by small lymphocytes. Also, an inflammatory process takes place at the junction of graft and the recipient body. The drugs used by surgeons and their medical teams to control graft rejection are primarily drugs which prevent cell division; their effectiveness in preventing the rejection of grafts is presumably achieved by preventing the small lymphocytes that have been triggered by the foreign antigens from proliferating. Other methods of controlling graft rejection concentrate on destroying large numbers of small lymphocytes; such methods are the use of whole-body irradiation and the use of antilymphocytic serum, which is the preparation of antibody specifically against lymphocytes. On the other hand, there are some experts who hold the view that prevention of inflammation would be the best way of securing the acceptance of a grafted organ.

I have presented in this chapter the latest views about how the immune processes actually work. The question of what prevents my immune system from attacking antigens on my own cells, antigens which cause the immune system of, say, a sheep to react very strongly, has gone unanswered but will be dealt with when we come to consider auto-immune diseases. I am declared to be "tolerant" of my own antigens, unless I have auto-immune disease, but how can I be made "tolerant" of someone else's antigens if I need an organ transplant? What happens if I am "tolerant" to cells which it would be best if I rejected—is this what happens when I get cancer? Is the immune system also a "police force" against subversion in my own body's cells? All these problems will be dealt with in appropriate chapters later. For the moment I want to look back and see the paths by which immunology has reached the state of understanding I have just described.

Chapter 4

The Early History of the Science

The history of immunology is a glorious example of the success of the "suck it and see" method. Immunology was successful long before anyone even knew of the existence of the germs and organisms against which it provided protection. Millions of lives were saved, untold epidemics and suffering avoided, long before any sound theoretical base of understanding was achieved. If anyone still believes that science proceeds by careful observation of phenomena, followed by the enunciation of a basic law of nature which can only be applied to bring about further advances when the phenomena are fully understood, then immunology is a living disproof of that theory. Immunology has been used successfully by men attempting to reproduce a natural phenomenon which they little understood.

It all began, it seems, with the Chinese and the Arabs, who observed, many centuries ago, that a person who had recovered from an attack of smallpox rarely seemed to contract the disease again. Thucydides noted that during the plague of Athens (whatever disease that may have been), only those few who had recovered from the disease were able to nurse the sick and bury the dead. In other words, the phenomenon of immunity was widely known. It was most probably the Chinese and the Arabs who first converted that observation into a clinical treatment by actually infecting people with material from the pustules of smallpox victims in the attempt to produce immunity artificially by giving a mild attack of the disease. This treatment was of particular value to young girls who thus might escape the pockmarks of a more serious attack. Voltaire, the cynic, attributes the development of smallpox immunisation entirely to the combination of female vanity and male lust; he claims that the practice was carried on principally by the Circassians, who had virtually no other exportable asset than the beauty of their daughters. "In order therefore to preserve the life and beauty of their children the thing remaining was to give them the smallpox in their infant years," he writes in his *Letters*. "This they did by inoculating in the body of the child, a pustule taken from the most regular, and at the same time the most favourable sort of smallpox that could be procured."

Technically this practice of inoculation with human smallpox material should be called variolation, from the name of the organism, "variola." The practice was brought to England by a remarkable woman, Lady Mary Wortley Montagu, wife of the British Ambassador in Constantinople, who had her own son treated in this way during her stay in the Ottoman capital. When she returned to London in 1718 she made a determined attempt to convert her fellow countrymen to the same practice. There was certainly fertile soil for her preaching, since a contemporary medical writer recorded that "three score persons in every hundred have the smallpox. Of these three score, twenty die of it in the most favorable season of life, and as many more wear the disagreeable remains of it in their faces so long as they live." A twentieth-century writer, John Rowan Wilson, has described how Lady Mary "became the first to experience the emotional atmosphere which seems to be a characteristic response to any ex-

periments in immunisation. The clergy thundered at her
from the pulpits for proposing to tamper with the designs of
Providence and she was accused of being an unnatural
mother for experimenting with her own children." [1]

Lady Mary Wortley Montagu was, however, a strong
character, and what was more important, an influential person in the days when being an aristocrat really meant having
power (on both sides of the Atlantic). The new practice was
first tested on six condemned criminals in Newgate Gaol. Or-
phan children of St. James's Parish in London were the next
experimental subjects. The real triumph came when Princess
Caroline had two of the royal daughters inoculated. From
then onwards the practice of inoculation spread. "One Royal
infant in 1718 was worth as much for the purpose of proof
as several hundred thousand ordinary children in 1956.
. . . In those days also there was no one to question the as-
sumption that human lives carried different degrees of
value." [2]

Cynicism apart, variolation spread rapidly in Britain
and Western Europe. It has been suggested that its ability to
prevent the deaths especially of young people and of women
of child-bearing age was a major factor in the great increase
in population which occured in Britain in the first half of the
eighteenth century, and which was in itself an essential preliminary to the coming of the Industrial Revolution and the
urban civilisation in which we now live. But, of course, variolation had its own death rate, by no means negligible; it
was a highly dangerous procedure and the material used in
the inoculation was quite capable of starting an epidemic of
smallpox. So the search for a safer material began.

The first recorded instance of the use of cowpox virus to
achieve immunity against smallpox came in Dorsetshire in
southwest England in 1774. A local farmer, Benjamin Jesty,
inoculated his own wife in the arm under the elbow with a

needle, having obtained his material "on the spot from the cows of Farmer Elford of Chittenhall."

It was a widespread belief among country people at that time that cowpox, if caught from cows by man, protected him against smallpox. Edward Jenner, a Gloucestershire physician, heard this piece of local lore from a country-woman and spent several years investigating the possibility before he tried his crucial experiment in 1796.

Jenner's great experiment was one that we would today consider unacceptable ethically. It was heroic, at least as far as the experimental "animal" was concerned. This was one James Phipps, an eight-year-old boy of whose previous and subsequent history we know nothing. Jenner, using a lancet, took infected material from the pustule of a milkmaid who had caught cowpox and then immediately made scratches on the arm of the boy with the blade of the same lancet. In a few days the boy developed fever and a headache, and a pus-tule appeared at the scratched place on his arm. The fever and symptoms quickly subsided, however, and the pustule, after appearing as a small ulcer for a few days, quietly healed up—exactly the reaction in James Phipps that we are all accustomed to nowadays when we are vaccinated. But this of itself proved nothing. James Phipps had to demon-strate his immunity to smallpox when Jenner tried to infect him, six weeks later, with material from a smallpox patient. Fortunately for both Jenner and Phipps, the immunity had been established and the practice of vaccination had been given an experimental basis. It is called vaccination because the basic disease material came from the cow, which in Latin is called *vacca*.

Follow-up experiments and treatment were not immedi-ately possible because the local epidemic of cowpox waned and Jenner was unable to obtain any more material until the disease started up again in the cattle two years later. But in

1798 Jenner was able to start work again, and he was also
able to develop his technique by vaccinating fresh patients
with material taken from patients whose pustules he had
himself caused by earlier vaccinations. His work was very
largely successful, but as the knowledge spread, so did the
controversy. In 1798 Jenner published his first pamphlet:
"An Inquiry into the Causes and Effects of the Variolae Vac-
ciniae." He believed that cowpox was really no more than a
slight or less virulent form of smallpox, and his pamphlet, in
the words of John Rowan Wilson, "set a pattern of over-
optimism which has persisted with occasional exceptions to
the present day." [3]

Despite fierce opposition, Jenner's work and position
gained strength. He secured Court patronage; the medical
profession of those days largely accepted his conclusions
when seventy of the leading physicians and surgeons in London made a public declaration endorsing his thesis. It is estimated that 100,000 people had been vaccinated by 1800.
Learned societies in Britain and Europe offered Jenner
honors and decorations—though not the Royal College of
Physicians, which insisted that he pass an examination in
Classics before he could be admitted to membership. But
Jenner believed, and stated publicly, that a person once vaccinated could never catch smallpox—a foolish pronounce-
ment, entirely unjustified by modern scientific standards,
which was to bring his whole cause into disrepute.

For several years the death rate from smallpox in Britain
and Western Europe did fall dramatically. But then it
started to rise again and there were a number of well-
founded reports of cases of smallpox even among the vaccinated. Jenner refused to abandon his position, and defended
it in a stream of publications, some of which were distinctly
bizarre in tone. But when he died, those less emotionally involved were realising that the answer to the problem was

repeated revaccination—at least as a practical measure. No one seems to have had the least inkling, as the first conquest of an infectious disease in the history of mankind got under way, of why the campaign against smallpox was succeeding. The theoretical knowledge—the acknowledgement that invisible organisms, germs, were the cause of infectious diseases—had to wait for almost exactly one hundred years after the first successful attempts by Jenner to protect a human being against disease by increasing, artificially, his immunity to that disease.

Immunology as a science, rather than as an uncomprehended but practical treatment, began in 1877. It was originated in Paris by Louis Pasteur.

Pasteur a few years earlier had founded the sciences of biochemistry and bacteriology by showing in his work on the problems of brewing that both infection and fermentation were the results of the activity of living organisms. Pasteur not only discovered the existence of germs and opened the way to the discovery of the whole range of micro-organisms; he was above all the first scientist in medicine, the founder of modern medical science. And because we regard Pasteur as the founder of so many scientific disciplines and lines of clinical practice which are beneficial to us, we forget how much of a shock he delivered to humanity. It was Pasteur who showed us a whole range of creatures—a whole set of nucleic acid groupings—competing with us for possession of the earth's surface; a discovery just as shocking to human susceptibilities as would be the discovery of the invasion of our earth by invisible creatures from outer space.

Pasteur was not medically qualified as a doctor. He therefore had to do most of his work with the animals normally used in veterinary practice. Very shortly after his successful establishment of the germ theory, in fact, in 1877, when he was fifty-five years old, he turned to immunology. He was desperately keen to show that the germ theory could be used for practical purposes. "It seemed to Pasteur, as to a great many others, that immunity was a general phenomenon related to most infectious diseases, and that there should theoretically be some means of preparing a variety of vaccines for various conditions," says Wilson.[4]

Pasteur was naturally interested in the bacteria he had himself discovered: he was interested to know what they were and he was interested in the new forms then being rapidly discovered by other scientists following his lead. But his primary concern was to obtain practical applications from the rapidly developing knowledge of microbes. There is a story told by one of his colleagues, who rather cautiously explained to the great man that a microbe, which Pasteur had described as a "coccus," was in reality a very small member of the different family of "bacilli." After a terrifying pause Pasteur is reputed to have said: "If you only knew how little difference that makes to me."

The basic problem at hand before immunology could begin was to find a method by which the antigen could be introduced into the body without producing the full-scale disease (to use our modern terminology). Jenner's success was based on centuries of human observation. It had been spotted that cowpox produced the effect of artificial immunity against smallpox, which, as we now say, means that the vaccinia virus carries antigens either the same as or sufficiently like the antigens of smallpox/variola to produce the effects of immunity. What Pasteur had to do, since the artificial synthesis of antigens was as yet inconceivable, was to find either analogues of all infectious organisms, as cowpox is the analogue of smallpox, or some way by which normally infectious and virulent organisms could be turned into avirulent, harmless creatures which nevertheless still retained the antigenic specificity of the virulent germs.

The way he achieved success is one of the classic "happy accident" stories of science, though much less well known than the story of Fleming and penicillin which it so much resembles. Pasteur was working with chicken cholera bacillus, and he had a strain of the bacillus which invariably caused death to chickens when injected even in minute amounts. But during a summer vacation some of the cultures of the chicken cholera bacillus were left lying around for a few weeks—this was in the days before laboratory refrigeration.

When he injected some of these older cultures into chickens, the birds did not die. It is the mark of the great scientist that he has the intuition to know when the accident or the unusual result is significant. Pasteur followed up his apparent mistake in technique by preparing fresh cultures of chicken cholera bacillus. But when he gave these fresh cultures, in the crucial experiment, to the chickens who had received the "worn-out" culture, they still did not die—they had been immunised.

Thus the phenomenon of "attenuation" had been discovered. Attenuation means that a change in the organism is produced so that it can still grow and multiply, and possesses the same external antigenic shapes or determinants, but is less lethal, less virulent, less dangerous. Pasteur soon discovered that the exposure to light and changes of temperature which had affected his culture of chicken cholera bacillus and attenuated the strain of bacteria involved was by no means the most efficient way of achieving attenuation. Prolonged culture under airless conditions had the same effect. And then he was able to show that attenuation could also be achieved with anthrax germs. He conducted a famous public experiment at Pouilly-le-Fort, where he showed that attenuated anthrax germs provided immune protection to nearly all the experimental animals (twenty-four sheep, one goat, and six cattle) when they were challenged with a particularly virulent anthrax bacillus which killed most of the control (non-immunised) animals.

He then discovered attenuation by "passaging," which is the usual means by which the modern pharmaceutical industry produces vaccines. It involves injecting a culture of organisms into some animal not normally affected by the disease. Nowadays, this is usually the laboratory mouse, rat, or rabbit; for Pasteur it was pigs, pigeons, or rabbits. Infective material is recovered from the body of the animal and injected into yet another of the same species. After many such "passages," often accompanied by considerable dilutions of the number of organisms in the injection at each passage, an avirulent strain can usually be recovered.

This process of attenuation by passaging does not necessarily involve the scientist in ever isolating or discovering the infective organism itself. Pasteur certainly lacked the equipment and technology to isolate or identify a virus—a task right at the limit of our present technology, using the electron microscope. But he could produce successful vaccines against virus diseases. It is fascinating to realise that the first two human diseases to be successfully treated by immunisation, smallpox and rabies, are both virus diseases—diseases caused by "organisms" (though many would dispute that a virus is an organism), which were not even known to exist for half a century after Pasteur had first discovered the existence of bacteria.

But Pasteur was certainly able to attenuate the rabies virus by passaging it from one rabbit brain to another and finally by cultivating the virus in the spinal cords of rabbits, which were then hung up to dry for at least two weeks. He showed that emulsions made from this dried rabbit spinal cord protected dogs from virulent rabies virus and also from infection transmitted by the saliva of rabid street dogs. Furthermore, his rabies vaccinations gave protection even if they were started after the dog had received a dose of infective material; rabies virus travels very slowly along the nerve fibres before multiplying in the brain and spinal cord cells, and is not found in the blood stream—hence the extremely long incubation period for rabies.

The moment for the great transfer of Pasteur's skill and discoveries from animal to human patients came when a small boy from Alsace, Joseph Meister, was brought to Pasteur. The boy had been bitten many times by a dog that was undoubtedly rabid. Pasteur started the course of thirteen injections of emulsified rabbit spinal cord material three days after the boy had been bitten; the boy survived and ended his days as gate-keeper at the Institut Pasteur in Paris.

These were Pasteur's triumphs. It was the founding of modern scientific immunology. But before Pasteur was dead the controversies had started. The basis of the attacks on immunology was the simple, but inescapable, fact that it is impossible to prove scientifically that an immunisation has worked, in the sense of definitely preventing an attack of the disease in any individual case. Nowadays, we can prove the presence of antibody in the vaccinated animal where none or very little was present before the immunisation, and statistically we can show the decrease of a disease in the face of a program of mass vaccination. This will satisfy us as to the practical value of immunisation, but it proves nothing for any individual. On the other hand, it is possible to prove with reasonable certainty in an individual case that a drug is responsible for a cure. In Pasteur's time a commission was set up to investigate his methods after the cure of Joseph Meister and the successful treatment of a number of other cases of human beings bitten by rabid dogs. The commission found in Pasteur's favour and set up a service available for all suspected cases of rabies.

It did not stop people from saying that Pasteur's vaccine had killed the patient in cases where the patient died, and maintaining that the patients had not been infected with rabies anyway when they survived. And a huge problem arises with all vaccines made from attenuated strains of infective organisms, the so-called live vaccines: the danger that the attenuated strain may spontaneously revert to its original virulence or at least to a more virulent form. This has meant that live vaccines have, on the whole, been limited to veterinary purposes until the last thirty years. With the original exceptions of smallpox and rabies most human vaccines have not been of the live type. (The live polio vaccine was the first major change in this situation; since then, the new measles and German measles vaccines introduced in the last three years have also been live vaccines.) Most people nowadays reject so automatically Lady Mary Wortley Montagu's idea of trying out a new vaccine on orphans and condemned criminals, including the necessary check on the efficacy of the vaccine by challenging them with the real disease, that it is difficult to realize what a problem this presents for the medical scientist. The obvious method of proving the case just cannot be applied on ethical grounds.

Pasteur himself had no idea of the science of self or that it was the body's ability to recognise not-self that made his treatments successful. Naturally, he could see that immunisation brought some important change in the body of the animal, but he had only one idea as to what that change might be. It was published in 1880. Then, very vaguely and tentatively, he put forward a hypothesis that some foodstuff necessary for the survival of the dangerous germ in the body was used up by the preliminary immunisation. But the "exhaustion theory" was soon forced out of the field by the rapidly growing amount of research being done by other scientists who rushed into the newly opened fields of bacteriology, microbiology, and immunology. It soon became plain that some very positive, active contribution by the host-body was necessary to explain immunisation.

It was work in the Institut Pasteur in 1888 that primarily killed the exhaustion theory and at the same time opened the way to the next major developments in immunology. This was the demonstration by Pierre Roux and Alexandre Yersin that if a culture of diphtheria bacilli was filtered in such a way that no bacteria could get through, the poison (toxin) produced by the bacilli was still present in the filtrate and the body could be made immune to the toxin alone. A flood of new discoveries followed, many of them emanating from the institute in Berlin where Robert Koch was the great figure. The technical basis of the advances made by Koch and his colleagues were his improvements in microscope techniques, and particularly the methods of straining microorganisms with various dyes so that they could be seen and, indeed, identified often according to the stains they absorbed.

By 1890 it had been shown that the immunity against a toxin only (i.e., without the originating micro-organism) was due to the production by the body of a substance which neutralized the toxin. It could further be shown that this antitoxin was specific to the toxin produced by that particular micro-organism. It was subsequently shown that the antitoxin made by one individual animal could be transferred to another and the second animal thus made immune to that particular toxin. In modern jargon, immunity can be passively conferred.

Another great figure of German nineteenth-century science, Paul Ehrlich, then demonstrated that the body could also manufacture antitoxin against poisons which were not produced by micro-organisms. He demonstrated that the blood serum could quickly acquire the power to neutralize injections of ricin, an extract of castor oil that is highly poisonous and often lethal.

The word "antibody" had been coined before antibodies were definitely proved to exist. The person who succeeded in proving this was another German, Richard Pfeiffer, in 1894 when he was studying the organisms which cause cholera, the cholera vibrios. All this tied in with the earlier discovery (1886) by Salmon and Theobald Smith, using chicken cholera bacilli like Pasteur, that injections of dead bacilli could also give immunity in certain cases. They had killed their bacilli by heat, and had thus founded the line of vaccines which depend on the use of "killed" organisms (like the Salk polio vaccine which preceded the Sabin "live" polio vaccines). The essence of the killed vaccine is that the organisms retain their antigenic structure sufficiently to prime the immune system, although they are incapable of multiplying and causing damage. And, in fact, the concept of antigen as the opposite of antibody was first voiced at this time, in the 1890's. However, theories were not of great interest in the rush of practical achievements, and laboratory technology was not sufficient to allow any further definition of the theories of antibody and antigen.

Nonetheless, the actions of antibody as shown by Pfeiffer did have two important features, in addition to the general function of neutralising micro-organisms and their toxins. These features were agglutination, the action of antibody in clumping together bunches of micro-organisms or cells, and precipitation, the result of antibody combining with cells or macromolecules so as to give a visible precipitate in a culture fluid.

The tests using agglutination or precipitation have steadily become more and more important. If, for instance, a passenger on a plane from Bombay is taken ill and smallpox is suspected, we can test for the presence of variola in his blood long before the symptoms on his body become decisive, by testing samples of his blood against the serum of a horse which has been injected with smallpox material many months before and which must therefore contain antibodies to smallpox. And this sort of technique has become even finer: we can, for example, rapidly establish the precise family grouping of common germs such as diphtheria or streptococci by taking material from the patient and testing it against the various antibodies developed by laboratory animals against all the known types of the germ in question.

The first great era of immunology came to an end in 1894, when Roux announced that serum from an immunised horse would cure patients suffering from diphtheria. It immediately raised the possibility that a wide variety of other diseases could be cured by providing the sufferers with antibodies preformed against the germ in animals. The hope proved illusory, for in no other disease has serum proved so effective as in diphtheria, though the antitoxin made by horses against tetanus toxin has proved very useful as a prophylactic treatment in cases of large open wounds.

But in essence all the weapons of practical immunology for the next fifty years had been discovered by 1894—the live attenuated vaccine and the killed vaccine, both of which encouraged the body to manufacture its own antibody against the specific invading organism or damaging toxin—and the provision of preformed antibody from another creature, which is the essence of serotherapy. The early experiences with these treatments taught some essential, and slightly deflating, lessons. These were that even natural immunity does not necessarily last for a lifetime, that vaccination with live vaccines lasts longest among the artificially induced immunities, while vaccination with killed vaccine may give immunity for only a short period of a year or two, and that passively conferred immunity may well last only for a period of months.

Cholera was a great scourge of the slums of Western European cities throughout the nineteenth century, and the development of cholera vaccines well illustrates the development of immunology in the great early days of the practical use of the new science. The first cholera immunisations, by using live attenuated organisms, proved far too dangerous an experiment for any major program to be launched.

However, a slight variation on the original technique of killing cholera vibrios by heat to produce a killed vaccine—killing them with the chemical phenol—allowed a vaccine to be produced which gave immunity for a year or so. But reimmunisation every six months was necessary for complete safety, and it was obvious that a large population could not be expected to turn up voluntarily at such short intervals. The vaccine was therefore good for use only in face of an epidemic, and this is the way we use it nowadays, or for travellers who must pass briefly through an area where cholera is rife. Meanwhile, the disease has been virtually wiped out in Western cities, not by an immunisation program but by the provision of proper sewage and clean water supplies.

There was a rather similar experience with typhoid. A short-lasting immunity given by a killed vaccine became available before 1900. But as soldiers can easily be paraded and compelled to have regular revaccinations, the vaccine was widely used in the Boer War and in most military campaigns since. Much later, in 1940, a killed vaccine against typhus was developed.

The major attempt in the first decades of the present century to produce a live vaccine was the development of an anti-tuberculosis vaccine. This was called B-C-G, because the attenuated strain of the mycobacterium that causes tuberculosis had been discovered by two Frenchmen and was named after them—Bacille Calmette-Guérin. B-C-G was in fact the first live bacterial vaccine to be used on a large scale in man, but its wide acceptance was delayed by a catastrophe in Germany when a batch of the vaccine was found to be contaminated. Experience has proved that vaccines based on this attenuated strain of tubercle bacilli are, in fact, safe and there have been extensive campaigns to immunise schoolchildren in Britain and most West European countries since 1950.

The greatest success of the immunologists in the first half of this century lies almost certainly in the virtual elimination of diphtheria from our childhood. The important discovery here was made by Glenny in 1923, when he found that careful treatment of toxins, including diphtheria toxin, with formaldehyde destroyed their dangerous potential without affecting their antigenicity or immunising capacity. Within the following ten years a safe vaccine using this "toxoid" was prepared and, led by the example of the town of Hamilton, in Ontario, Canada, a number of mass vaccination campaigns has succeeded in almost completely eliminating diphtheria from the industrialized or developed nations. As a qualification it must be added, however, that there is evidence that the diphtheria germs which are still found in few, but regularly occurring, cases, seem to be much less virulent than the strains that were known in the 1920's. There is similar evidence of loss of virulence in scarlatina (scarlet fever) germs.

All these immunological successes of the fifty years from 1890 to 1940 were achieved against bacteria and other microorganisms of the same sort of size. These are all organisms that are fully formed cellular creatures, capable of autonomy, of living by themselves in nutrient cultures, i.e., broths and jellies containing the substances they need for nutrition. The viruses present different problems. Because of their very small size they cannot really be seen except under the electron microscope; even more seriously, they cannot live by themselves—they must enter a living cell and use its mechanisms for their own reproduction and multiplication. This means that viruses cannot be kept for study in the laboratory except in living infected animals. But all animals, even the laboratory mouse, are comparatively expensive to keep and difficult to handle. Progress with viruses was therefore slow.

It is true that Karl Landsteiner managed to give monkeys polio in 1908 and Theiler gave yellow fever to mice in 1928. Thus some progress in studying at least the effects of the virus could be made. It was not established that influenza was a virus disease until Wilson Smith managed to give ferrets influenza in 1933. And at about that time, in 1931 to be precise, Goodpasture showed how to cultivate virus in "chick embryos," more commonly known as hens' eggs. The hen egg provides a sterile environment in which the virus can multiply for study without contamination and it is at the same time cheap and easy to handle. But real progress against viruses had to wait until the invention of tissue-culture techniques—that is, the breeding of viruses in collections of living cells which are themselves kept alive in the test tube by providing them with nutrient fluid. The arrival of antibiotics made this possible, by keeping the cells free from unwanted infection and the virus free from contamination by bacterial growths. Chick-embryo culture had, however, allowed the development of vaccines against fowl pest, hog cholera, and Rocky Mountain spotted fever, as well as the development of a better rabies vaccine, based on virus grown in duck eggs. (Pasteur's rabies vaccine had always carried the danger of giving the recipient encephalitis from rabbit nerve tissue; this could not be separated from the virus which had grown on it.)

The last great vaccine to be produced before the middle of this century was yellow fever immunisation. Yellow fever had prevented de Lesseps from building the Panama Canal as well as the Suez Canal. It nearly stopped the Americans from building the Canal, too, in the years just before the

First World War. It was control of mosquitoes by a continuous spraying of every ditch and puddle where they could breed that kept the sickness figures from malaria and yellow fever down at least to a level where the engineering could carry on. Only in 1927 and 1928, at last, the first signs of progress against yellow fever could be seen when the disease was successfully given to Rhesus monkeys and mice. But it was dangerous work; Stokes and Noguchi were killed by the disease they were trying to control. The French developed the Dakar strain of attenuated organism and from this they manufactured a vaccine. But many people considered the Dakar strain vaccine to be still dangerous, and Theiler in particular, who, working in the United States, had successfully infected mice with yellow fever. He pursued his own line of work and eventually, in 1936, produced the attenuated 17D strain that has become the standard yellow fever vaccine for most of the world.

This chapter has developed into something frighteningly like a canter through the history of the conquest of infectious disease. What I want to emphasise rather is the fact that all this achievement came about without any real understanding of how immunity worked. It was known that antibodies were produced by the body in response to invasion by microorganisms, toxins, large organic molecules, and even to perfectly bland and innocuous substances so long as the molecules were large enough. But how, or by what, the antibodies were produced was quite unknown; still less was it known how specific antibodies were produced, though it was quite clear that the antibodies were highly specific. Indeed, Landsteiner had used the specificity of antibodies as early as 1900 to show that there were at least three main blood groups in man, the familiar A, B, and O. In fact, no one even knew how antibodies neutralized the invaders, and the biggest controversy of all surrounded one simple question: How did the

immune system cope with invading micro-organisms? The
majority of the evidence in the last twenty years of the nineteenth century seemed to point to "humoral" factors, that is,
substances circulating in the blood stream, as the body's
chief defensive weapons. But there was at least one great advocate of a different view: that the immune response was
largely a matter of action by cells.

Even severe textbooks allow themselves to use the word
"rumbustious" to describe Eli Metchnikoff, a Russian born
near Kharkov in 1845, who studied zoology and embryology
at the universities of Kharkov and St. Petersburg. He then
worked in various jobs at various places. Indeed, his career
could be described as typical of a biologist; in 1882 he was a
professor at the University of Messina and resigned in an up-
roar, the cause of which is unknown. Without a job, but
equally without loss of nerve, Metchnikoff carried on, in his
own words, "indulging enthusiastically in researches in the
splendid setting of the Straits of Messina."

Then, one day when his family had gone to a circus,

> I remained alone at my microscope observing the life in the
> mobile cells of a transparent starfish larva, when a new
> thought suddenly flashed across my brain. It struck me that
> similar cells might serve in the defence of the organism against
> intruders. Feeling that there was in this something of surpass-
> ing interest, I felt so excited that I began striding up and
> down the room and even went to the seashore to collect my
> thoughts. I said to myself that if my supposition was true, a
> splinter introduced into the body of a starfish larva, devoid of
> blood vessels or of a nervous system, should soon be sur-
> rounded by mobile cells as is to be observed in a man who
> runs a splinter into his finger.

Metchnikoff immediately fetched a few rose thorns and introduced them under the skin of some of his starfish larvae.
By the following morning he found that experiment had con-

firmed his theory: "That experiment formed the basis of the phagocyte theory to the development of which I devoted the next twenty-five years of my life." [5]

Basing himself at the Institut Pasteur in Paris, Metchnikoff did indeed spend many years in furious controversy with the great German scientists of his day. He admitted that various soluble factors in blood serum plainly must play a part in acquired immunity. But since exposure to serum alone did not kill bacteria, there was, consequently, an important role to be played by cells, notably phagocytes, in innate immunity (what we now call non-specific immunity). In his studies—which were more what we nowadays think of as comparative physiology than immunology—he showed that in evolutionary terms the phagocytes seemed to be behaving exactly like primitive amoeba, in which the destruction of a potential invader and feeding itself are the same function. In more complicated but still primitive creatures like sponges the digestive process is likewise phagocytic in character, and phagocytes are named after their function of eating or ingesting material. In studying the relationship between the water flea, Daphnia, and the spores of a primitive fungus, Metchnikoff showed that the resistance of the flea, and indeed its survival, depended directly on the success of its phagocytes; if they failed, the flea died.

The controversy was settled by the man who conquered typhoid, Sir Almroth Wright. He proposed that the main action of the antibodies and other humoral factors was to help the phagocytes in their destruction of the invaders. In a sense, this is the modern view of the relationship between the humoral factors and the phagocytes, but we now know that there is a great deal more to the immune response than simple cooperation between antibody and phagocytes, which by the way are also numbered among the white cells or leucocytes.

Wright also was led to give the phagocytes too important a role. He is the original of Sir Colenso Ridgeon in Shaw's play, *The Doctor's Dilemma*, in which his doctrines were summed up: "There is at bottom only one genuinely scientific treatment of all diseases, and that is to stimulate the phagocytes. Stimulate the phagocytes. Drugs are a delusion." This may be poetic licence, but certainly Sir Almroth Wright is on record as having favoured attempts "to mobilize the immunological garrisons," and he used vaccination not just as a preventive treatment but also as a general method of treating infection. He would determine the type of organism responsible for a local infection, culture it, kill it, and inject the result back into the patient as an "autovaccine." He was also led into championing the cause of "laudable pus" in surgical wounds during the healing process—holding that the pus showed that the white corpuscles were active at the site. And since the antiseptics of those days could be shown to kill both bacteria and leucocytes at the same time, he held that antiseptics in infected wounds did no good and very probably some harm.

I digress, but it is interesting to remember that Sir Alexander Fleming discovered penicillin while working at St. Mary's Hospital in Paddington, London, under Sir Almroth Wright. One reason why the development of antibiotics took so long after their first discovery may well have been that an atmosphere of "Stimulate the phagocytes. Drugs are a delusion" can hardly have been intellectually conducive to the development of a new type of chemotherapy. Anyhow, the institute where they both worked is now named after the two of them.

Sir Almroth Wright wrote the article on Immunity in the fourteenth edition of the Encyclopaedia Britannica, published in 1929. A great deal of the article is in fact taken up with his compromise solution of the problem set by the opposing forces of the German "humoral factors" and Metchnikoff's phagocytic theory. Much of the rest seems extraordinarily old-fashioned although it was written only forty years ago, but it is quite clear that already the basic problem of the science of self had been grasped, though no acceptable answer was anywhere in sight. Wright quotes Ehrlich at considerable length, musing thus:

> If I take a guinea pig—that is a creature whose country of origin is Southern America—and administer to it abrin—a poison derived exclusively from Africa (and thus one which neither the tame guinea pig nor its ancestry can ever have encountered) and if I now find that my guinea pig furnishes me with an antidotal substance which indentures with the abrin as does a key with the wards of a lock for which it is made, is there then for me any way of escape from the conclusion that the organism of my guinea pig has specially constructed an antidotal substance to fit the particular kind of poison I have administered—performing in this a feat of chemical analysis and synthesis which would balk the ablest chemist?

Ehrlich correctly concluded that the only possible answer was that there must exist in the animal, already formed, some "receptor" molecules which would fit any introduced poison, and he correctly theorised, too, that the fitting of poison and receptor was a fitting together of molecules in three-dimensional shapes. But of lymphocytes there is no mention, and of the role of entire cells in immunity, except as phagocytes, there is not even speculation. Incidentally, Wright never uses the word "antibody," although he accepts that "counterpart substances" are manufactured by white blood cells.

Just as Ehrlich, one of the greatest scientists of all time, had posed the right question, the most difficult question, so many of his German colleagues had glimpsed what we now believe are roughly the right answers to many of the problems of immunology. Leo Loeb, for instance, published a very large book in 1910 entitled *The Biological Basis of Individuality*. This work actually suggested that lymphocytes were the cells which in some way examined the individuality of antigens presented to them. In that period, between 1890 and 1910, German immunologists had done autografts, that is, removing a piece of skin or part of some organ and replacing it in a different part of the owner's body. They had even performed a kidney transplant in a dog by 1905, and they had discovered that homografts, grafts between two different animals of the same species, would not work as a treatment. Ehrlich himself had suggested the "horror autotoxicus" as something which was not possible, and had thus in some sense seen at least the possibility of auto-immune disease.

From 1910 onwards, German science in general fell from its position of supremacy. This was, as we all know, largely due to political pressures: first, the anti-intellectualism of the Prussian spirit as the madness of the First World War gained hold; later, the specifically anti-scientific trend of Nazi thinking. But more important than the political pressures of twentieth-century Germany in bringing this promising line of scientific thought to a halt was the fact that scientific, laboratory technology was not available to provide experimental support for these speculations and exploratory grafting techniques. There were no electron microscopes for the close study of cells and viruses; there were no antibiotics to keep tissue cultures and surgical wounds free from infection. Quite as important was the necessity to await parallel developments in other scientific disciplines. It was difficult or even impossible to imagine, to hypothesise about, the linking and binding of antigen and antibody without the background of general knowledge of the three-dimensional structure of molecules which is nowadays provided by stereo-chemistry and molecular biology. Similarly, without our present knowledge of the structure of chromosomes and of the nucleic acids which make them up, it was difficult even to speculate on the possible answers to what seemed impossible dilemmas. If Ehrlich had known that the genes of his South American guinea-pig were made of the same basic material as the genes of his African poison-producing plant, he might well have seen many possible answers to his problem. In fact, there was a forty-year gap between the ending of the great flowering of German immunology in 1910 and the start of modern immunology in Australia, America, and Britain in the early 1950's.

But the start of this modern era of immunology was masked from most people's view by the greatest triumph of the old-style "vaccinator," the development of polio vaccine.

Poliomyelitis, infantile paralysis, is a virus disease in which the virus attacks specifically the nerve cells, and most particularly the nerves controlling muscular action. It can cause death, but its more spectacular result is to leave its victims paralysed either totally or just in one particular limb, with muscle wasting following on the inability to use the limb or limbs affected. Polio differs from most of the other infectious diseases that have scourged mankind in that it has only come to our notice within the last one hundred years, "like concentration camps, Public Relations and bubble gum, it is a phenomenon of the twentieth century," says John Rowan Wilson.[6] In fact, the first definitely accepted epidemic of polio occurred in Sweden in 1887, when there were 44 known cases. The first large epidemic occurred in Vermont in 1894, with 119 cases, and in the 1916 American epidemic there were 27,000 cases, with 6,000 deaths. The worst-hit area was New York City.

We now understand why polio is a feature of our modern,

hygienic Western civilisation—it is because the infection, if acquired in childhood, usually is very slight, no more than a stomach upset, which many of us living today but born before the vaccine was developed undoubtedly had without our parents knowing. The disease affects most seriously those who get it in young adulthood; it is among this group that paralysis occurs most often. The scars of the disease, in the shape of paralysis of various intensities, these people carry with them throughout life in the midst of our society. The scars of polio are as obvious to us as the pockmarks of smallpox were two hundred years ago; but, worse than the pockmarks, they imply a partially ruined life.

In the infectious stages, polio virus is excreted in the faeces, so polio in its paralytic form is, in a roundabout way, the result of good drainage and proper plumbing. We noted earlier how young British soldiers and sailors often became victims of polio when they were stationed in Malta, where the vast majority of the population had encountered the virus in their babyhood and easily passed through the infection, becoming immune by the time they reached the dangerous age of young adulthood. The young servicemen had not encountered the germ in their childhood and were without any immunity to it when they came to a locality where it was in constant and normally harmless circulation. It was, then, hardly surprising that America, in which plumbing was so important a feature of life, should be hardest hit by polio.

Landsteiner had established, as far back as 1908, that polio was carried by a virus in a series of experiments in which he managed to transfer the disease to animals. But a number of attempts to find a treatment or prevention against the disease failed miserably. Vaccines prepared by Kolmer and Brodie in New York State failed completely when they came to trials in 1934. There was the Schultz treatment of 1936 and 1937, which consisted of spraying zinc sulphate up the nose; it blocked the ends of the olfactory nerves, which seemed to be one obvious entry point for the virus. The virus had never been located anywhere except in nerve cells, and it was believed at the time that it must travel along the nervous system to get at the spinal cord and motor nerves, where it then multiplied to cause paralysis. The treatment proved ineffective, however, in preventing polio, and since it was quite likely to destroy the sense of smell, even those most enthusiastic about it never launched a large-scale program. Similarly, the Retan treatment, which came to the fore in 1938 and which involved the infusion of saline solution, was soon declared a failure.

Meanwhile there was continuously in front of the eyes of the American people a President, Franklin Roosevelt, who was himself a victim of polio (contracted in 1921). The National Foundation for Infantile Paralysis was inaugurated in 1938, and this organisation remains to this day the most extraordinary example we have ever seen of enlisting public enthusiasm and support for the conquest of a single disease, and of raising enormous sums of money to finance research and special treatment centers all over the continent. Of course the Foundation has been criticised, chiefly by the medical profession, which deplored what seemed to many the unseemly ballyhoo and publicity attaching to research projects and trials they felt should be conducted in the decorous and unemotional atmosphere we like to think surrounds the truly scientific enterprise. But whereas most inoculations and vaccinations had up to then been concerned with diseases that, with the notable exception of diphtheria, many Westerners looked upon as rather exotic (smallpox, yellow fever, rabies, and typhoid, for instance), polio was a disease of the hometown, a disease of the bright warm days of the late summer and early fall. It was, too, a disease that struck particularly at the affluent, middle-class, and professional, rather than the poorer sections of the community. And the Foundation triumphed in the end—all those millions of dollars did lead to the conquest of polio.

But Roosevelt died, and for ten years there was no real progress to report. Not until 1949 did John Franklin Enders, an aloof and aristocratic New Englander, succeed in growing polio virus in a tissue culture of monkey kidney cells. At last the virus had reached the state where it could be studied and manipulated in the laboratory, without the expensive and all-too-often inconclusive and time-consuming use of relays of monkeys.

But before the end of 1949, another discovery proved less reassuring. Bodian and others, including the Australians under Sir Macfarlane Burnet, showed that there were three distinct types of polio virus, distinct antigenically and therefore distinct immunologically; thus, any polio vaccine would have to contain viruses of the three types to give full protection. But it was Bodian again, this time with Horstmann, who, three years later, detected virus in the blood stream and thus ended the belief that the virus both spread and multiplied entirely in the nervous system. This knowledge immediately enhanced the chances of a successful vaccine being found.

And it was in fact during the same year, 1952, that Jonas Salk began work on the methods of mass production of the "killed" vaccine he had been preparing and studying in the laboratory. The next year Salk performed his first experiments, naturally on a very small scale, in administering his killed vaccine to children.

At this stage the story varies from the traditional unfolding of the drama of scientific success. Because "meanwhile, in another part of the forest" an entirely different scientific group, led by the flamboyant Koprowski, was experimenting with an entirely different vaccine, a live attenuated vaccine.

The group was at work in the laboratories of the Lederle Company, one of the great pharmaceutical manufacturing companies of the world. The laboratories were situated, very pleasantly, on the banks of the Pearl River in Mississippi, and the strain of virus that Koprowski and his team were using was called the Pearl River strain.

Thus, in 1952–53 a number of elements with which the world of medical science and public health had never had to deal before were fused—and it was the clash of these elements that made the whole story of the polio vaccines such a traumatic experience. For the first time a major commercial conflict was imminent. There were two rival vaccines competing for a market consisting of virtually every child and most of the adults of the entire developed world. The decisions which the scientists, doctors, and public health officials would have to make were bound to be based on evidence of a statistical nature, and this evidence would have to be paraded before a mass audience, many of whom had little understanding of statistics though all had a passionate personal interest in the decisions to be made. For while it is easy enough to see an epidemic of smallpox ravaging an Indian city, and therefore comparatively easy to show that a drug or vaccination campaign is halting the progress of the infection, polio was unpredictable in its assaults. Some years were "good," others "bad," some places were affected, others were not.

Only by immense campaigns of vaccination covering hundreds of thousands of children could it be shown whether a vaccine was in fact effective.

This immediately brought up two complications. First, the administrative effort and scientific checking in such an enormous campaign would be extremely expensive and would require great cooperation and goodwill among both population and public health authorities; consequently, there would soon be a shortage of countries or populations among whom these vast trials could be carried out. Second, applying a live vaccine to great numbers of people presented incalculable dangers. How safe would such a vaccine be when applied on a scale previously unthought of? What were the risks of a return to virulence by the attenuated strain of virus? On the other hand, the killed vaccine, naturally safer, would not give such a long period of immunity, and could prove disastrous both financially and in terms of goodwill if a revaccination campaign had to be started shortly after the first campaign had ended.

The National Foundation for Infantile Paralysis, under its director, Basil O'Connor, who was himself a fund-raiser and organiser of genius rather than a scientist or doctor, plumped for speed and safety rather than long-term effectiveness. The Salk killed vaccine was put into production with several pharmaceutical firms towards the end of 1953. The first mass trial was started in April of 1954. It was a three-month campaign of vaccination, highly organized, statistically controlled; but the results could not be known for many months. It would probably take a full year before the effects, in terms of children not infected with polio, would become clear and could be scientifically assessed on a statistical basis. But if large numbers of children in the United States were to be protected before the "polio season" of 1955 started, they would have to be injected early in that year, that is, about the time the results of the mass trial would become available. If there was to be any large-scale use of the vaccine in 1955, industrial production of the vaccine would of necessity have to begin long, long before the results of the trial were known. O'Connor took the plunge and ordered, in 1954, 27 million doses of the vaccine for use in 1955. This meant that the trial in 1954 just *had* to show favourable results.

The results were announced on April 12, 1955, at Ann

Arbor, Michigan. There is no doubt that in the trial vaccinations of the early summer of 1954 the Salk vaccine did show a quite clear and satisfactory preventive effect against polio. It was the way the results were announced that offended so much medical and scientific opinion. Traditionally, and not entirely for reasons of academic snobbery, scientific results are published in a professional or academic journal, with full details of the methods used and the statistics produced. It is the essence of the scientific ethos and of the historical efficacy of science that results, together with full details of experimental methods, must be openly published. They can then be properly criticised, the experiment repeated by other laboratories, and the results thus confirmed or denied independently. The results of the first mass trial of the Salk vaccine, however, were announced at a nationally televised press conference, with the anxious eyes of the entire American nation watching to see if their particular scourge could be removed. And the results promised that the scourge would be removed.

The administration of those 27 million doses which had been ordered began immediately after the Ann Arbor press conference. Within three weeks disaster seemed to have struck. Before the end of that dramatic April, the first reports came in of cases of poliomyelitis which had occurred immediately after vaccination. For a few days it was possible to assume that these few cases were occurring because the unfortunate patients had actually been infected with natural polio before the vaccination. But as more reports came in during the first weeks of May it became clear that the vaccinations were in fact causing the polio. There could be only one explanation: the virus had not been properly killed in at least some of all those millions of industrially produced doses. The question was whether there was some inherent weakness in the process or whether there had been a failure

of the safety measures and quality control in one particular
industrial plant. Anguished but swift enquiries revealed that
in every case where the vaccine was suspected of causing the
disease, the injected material had come from one specific
manufacturer (Cutter).

After a terrible pause in June, increased safeguards in
manufacturing were introduced and the campaign was allowed to proceed. There was no failure of nerve and this per-
severance was justified, for no further cases of polio after
vaccination were reported and the vast campaign went
ahead. In the next year, 1956, there was a further massive
campaign in the United States and the Salk vaccine also
began to be used on a large scale in Canada and several European countries. The killed vaccine appeared to be a clear
winner.

For, meanwhile, Koprowski and Cox at Lederle were
making but slow progress with their live vaccine, one of the
difficulties being to achieve coverage against all three types
of polio. Another of their difficulties was to find areas in
which they could carry out mass trials. As the use of the Salk
vaccine spread so rapidly this became more and more of a
problem; indeed, by only 1958 Koprowski was carrying out
trials in the Congo, an area where the conditions were so
difficult that the results were necessarily open to criticism on
the grounds that control was virtually impossible. But even
before, in 1957, Professor Dick, of Queen's University, Bel-
fast, had published a report which openly criticised the live
vaccine. A World Health Organisation committee, which
had been considering the rival merits of the killed and live
vaccines, published a somewhat inconclusive report in that
same year. In the meantime, one country after another had
taken up the Salk vaccine.

Few people had noticed the strictly scientific report in
which a man named Sabin had announced some successful

results with a live attenuated vaccine on 133 men in 1956, the year of triumph for the Salk vaccine. Dr. Albert B. Sabin was very far from the American "folk" picture of the immigrant Jewish boy who made good. Of Russian-Jewish parents, working at the University Medical School in Cincinnati, naturally quiet and unobtrusive, he was essentially a "pure" scientist—a laboratory man who published his work only in the specialist scientific journals. (He is equally quiet and truly scientific to this day, though not so unobtrusive since he became president of the Weizmann Institute, the great Israeli centre of scientific research.) It came as something of a bombshell when in 1959 Sabin announced the results of successful large-scale trials of his live vaccine in Russia. The cold war was much colder in the 1950's, a fact which we tend to forget when we consider the unusual spectacle of an American scientist carrying out trials of a vaccine in Russia.

Koprowski and Cox, before this, had gone their separate ways. Koprowski's trial in the Congo in 1958 was regarded with some suspicion. Cox's trials in Berlin and Dade County, Florida, in 1960 turned up with very doubtful results and some hints of actual danger. In the same year an official arbitration in the United States came out in favour of the Sabin strains of attenuated virus; it was important at the time in that it gave measured scientific approval to the Sabin live strain. It was, however, the vast campaigns launched in Russia and the Communist East European nations for wholesale immunisation of their entire populations with this vaccine that finally turned the scale of world opinion; not that a counting of votes can decide a matter like this. It is a question of statistical numbers, in this case millions of people, successfully protected, multiplied by the number of years for which the protection lasts.

In 1961 doubts began to arise about the long-term effectiveness of the Salk vaccine. It had always been known that a killed vaccine gave a shorter period of immunity than a live vaccine, but for protection of a whole population over a period of decades a vaccine requiring continuous reinjection is at an obvious disadvantage over a single treatment. In fact, by 1962 the Sabin live vaccine had taken over the job of protection against polio. In that year the U.S.A. officially licensed the Sabin strains; Great Britain and most European countries likewise took the Sabin vaccine into regular use; in Russia and the Eastern European countries enormous and successful campaigns continued. As we all know now the Sabin vaccine was the eventual winner of the competition, and in so far as it was the first live vaccine to come into use for really large numbers of people, it represented more than just a commercial triumph. It was a major new step in immunological technology.

This work has been followed by live vaccines against measles and German measles, the former having appeared in 1969. It involved a fascinating comment on the improvements in safety and control. When a mass campaign of measles vaccination was started in Britain using two rival, commercially manufactured vaccines, it was possible to detect a difference in safety between the two when one was causing adverse reactions at the rate of 1 per million doses and the other at the rate of 1 in every half-million cases. The less safe of the two was withdrawn. In the case of the measles vaccine programs, too, there had been a killed vaccine in the race. After the world-wide experience with polio vaccines, the killed measles vaccine very rapidly fell out of wide favor as soon as it was plain that effective live vaccines were coming onto the market.

A mumps vaccine has recently been developed. It is in use in the U.S.A. but has not yet gained acceptance in all other countries where it has been developed. Nevertheless, it completes the possibility of vaccination against all the important widespread diseases of childhood. Influenza vaccines can also be made; many have been prepared, and in some countries they have been widely used. But because of the ability of the influenza virus to mutate into a new antigenic type so rapidly (it may be because influenza viruses can hybridize like plants), there is a perpetual race to catch up with the new mutants. Influenza spreads so rapidly round the world—Asian 'flu spread across the world during the late sixties in a few months—that a large program of industrial vaccine production against a new influenza type always seems likely to be defeated by the time factor. Immunisation of key personnel seems probably the best course every time a new mutant turns up, accompanied of course by immunisation of those most at risk from serious effects of the new 'flu, usually the very old and the very young.

Further ahead there may come vaccines against venereal disease, which is rapidly taking up a position as the most common infectious disease of the "developed" world. The recent discovery of a possible agent of infectious hepatitis (jaundice) opens up the prospect of developing a vaccine against this, too. But since it has not yet been shown that any human cancer or leukaemia has been caused by an infective agent, it is virtually pointless to speculate whether there will ever be an immunisation program aimed directly against cancer-causing viruses.

The crucial strategic feature of the development of live vaccines is that, because the live vaccine offers long-term, perhaps lifelong, immunity, it becomes possible to consider immunising the entire population of a modern nation or block of nations. Thus the virus in question can be knocked out of the life system for so long that it could completely cease to exist, unless it found another host population, perhaps among the birds, wild animals, or farm stock. If existence on the surface of our earth is indeed a struggle between different types of spiral molecules for the exclusive rights to use the other chemicals, then our type of molecule seems to have won a notable victory here. The chief qualification to this belief lies in wondering whether causing a fatal disease in an invaded organism can be to the evolutionary advantage of a virus, for by killing the living cells it needs in order to reproduce itself the virus would appear to be harming its long-term prospects. The ideal from a virus's point of view would seem to be to create a condition of subclinical infection, so that it can continue to parasitise its host without causing the total death of the host cells.

The development of the live vaccines in the last twenty years, while enormously important, has hardly added to the progress of immunology as the science of self. Although a genuine continuation of the older immunology, from the point of view of the development of immunological theory it is a digression. The crossroads in that development came when the discovery of antibiotics seemed to spell the end of immunology, and it is to this point in time that I now return.

Chapter 5

The Birth of the Theory of Self

The science of immunology reached its turning point in the five years immediately after the end of the Second World War, the years from 1945 to 1950. During this period it ceased to be simply a technology of preventive medicine and became instead a major discipline of science, with hypotheses that could be tested and confirmed or disproved, and applications very much wider than the mere prevention of infectious diseases. For this theoretical development opened the way to transplant surgery, to new ideas about cancer and possible ways of dealing with tumours, to new treatments for allergies, and life-saving methods of preventing such conditions as "Rhesus babies."

This sudden blooming of a new science came about largely because the old technology seemed virtually finished, at least from the point of view of intellectual development. The years of the war had seen intense activity on the part of the immunologists. They had been dragged from their laboratories and clinics and asked to cope with the medical problems posed by a world catastrophe, epidemics in armies and among huge masses of refugees, entire populations of displaced persons. They were asked to prepare protection against the influenza epidemics that were expected to sweep the world once the war was over, as they had swept the world after the First World War, killing more people than all the battles of 1914 to 1918. They were asked to protect soldiers fighting in the jungles of New Guinea and Burma, where few white men had ever penetrated before, as well as men fighting in African deserts and Arctic tundra. The most surprising thing is that they succeeded.

The Second World War differed from previous international conflicts in many ways, but perhaps the most important was that civilian casualties were very much higher than military casualties. One reason was that the Second World War was the first major conflict in which disease did not take more toll of the fighting forces than the enemy. This was not entirely owing to the work of the immunologists—the ability to control malaria with new drugs came much more from the chemists, and the advances in the techniques of blood transfusion saved many wounded who would have died in previous wars. But on the other hand, from 1941 on, typhus was controlled by vaccination, and many of the less dramatic, though equally casualty-producing, diseases like camp fever were controlled largely owing to the efforts of immunologists, even where no vaccine was produced. The immunologist was in any case prepared to deal with diseases like yellow fever, cholera, and typhoid, which had destroyed entire armies in previous campaigns.

Indeed, by the end of the war an American killed vaccine proved reasonably effective against influenza, so that attempts to produce live vaccines were dropped. A long-term campaign against the common cold was started in England shortly after the war. Only polio and the childhood diseases like measles and whooping cough seemed to be left as major targets for the immunologist.

Perhaps even more depressing for the morale of the scientists in immunology was the discovery of the antibiotics, beginning with penicillin, first manufactured on a large scale in the early 1940's. This was followed by a spate of "broad-spectrum" antibiotics shortly after the end of the war, when the big American pharmaceutical companies were able to divert their resources into the search for and development of new substances that would equal or surpass the action of penicillin. In those days, before we realised how effective the spread of bacterial resistance to antibiotics would be, it really seemed as though the problem of infectious disease had been overcome. To put it crudely, there was very little left for the immunologist to do, and not much intellectual excitement about that very little. "The old immunology just about died with the coming of antibiotics," according to Dr. John Humphrey. Humphrey admits that he only took on the leadership of the small immunology department being set up in those years by the Medical Research Council of Great Britain because he was a "scientific opportunist," and he felt that his work in pathology was not giving him final answers about anything and because he thought there were a few interesting leads into what might be the basic mechanism of immunology which others had barely noticed.

At the same time the excitement in the biological sciences was being generated in totally different fields. Biochemistry and a detailed study of genetics using bacteria laid the foundations for molecular biology. The build-up had started which was to lead to the Watson-Crick elucidation of the structure and mechanism of the genetic material of all living organisms, DNA (deoxyribonucleic acid). The view of life as a comprehensible physico-chemical system, which I tried to express in the opening paragraphs of this book as a struggle between competing spiral molecules, was beginning to enter human consciousness.

In one way, at least, this enormous surge of excitement

and discovery in the biological sciences, which has proved the most important intellectual advance of the last twenty years, had arisen from immunology. The progression from several purely immunological studies of disease-causing organisms to the realisation that the actual mechanism of genetics and heredity could be studied in the comparatively simple cases of bacteria by then-available laboratory techniques led to the possibility that a generalised understanding of genetic mechanisms could be obtained from the work of the bacterial geneticists. It is almost certainly true, however, that the present theories of the immunologists could not have arisen until the molecular biologists provided a system for understanding the chemical basis of heredity and the certainty that macromolecules work at least to some extent through their three-dimensional shape.

Many distinguished men and women have worked in these fields where bacterial genetics, molecular biology, biochemistry, and immunology now overlap, interact, and cross-fertilise each other. But the one most obvious link, the man whose life seems to connect them all most clearly, is once again the Australian, Sir Frank Macfarlane Burnet. There are good grounds for claiming that he was among the first to open up the possibility of studying bacterial genetics; he was awarded the Nobel prize for sharing in the discovery of immunological tolerance: His theory of clonal selection as the basis of the immune mechanism now seems triumphant, although in detail it has been changed from its original formulation.

The details of the origination of bacterial genetics are hardly of major importance for the story of immunology except in so far as they concern the story of this one man, and even in his life this subject plays only a small part. But in the early 1920's, when he was still a young doctor in charge of the clinical bacteriology of a Melbourne hospital, Macfarlane Burnet read about the discovery of bacteriophage by the Frenchman, d'Herelle, working at the Institut Pasteur in 1917. Bacteriophage, now more usually called just phage, are essentially viruses which infect bacteria. As they are so small and simple compared with living cellular systems of any sort, their mysteries are comparatively easy to unravel and they have been much used in deciphering the genetic code within the last five years. In the course of his laboratory duties Burnet was asked to examine a urine specimen, and he duly went through the process of sprinkling a few drops of the urine on a plate of agar (nutrient jelly) and incubating the plate. Next morning there was a typical, clearly visible growth of bacteria on the plate at all the points where the urine had dropped; the identification of the organism causing the patient's pyelitis was routine.

. . . but, much more interestingly, on the culture were two large perfectly typical bacteriophage clearings. It was easy enough to isolate the phage from one of those plaques, but that was unimportant. What impressed me was the fact that in all probability bacteriophage plaques (i.e. blank spaces in the culture where the virus has killed the growth of bacteria) must have been seen occasionally on urine cultures almost from the time when Koch first developed solid, jelly-like media for the growth of bacteria. No one however had apparently recognised that those clearings were significant and presented a phenomenon calling urgently for investigation. Even for an experienced scientist it is quite extraordinarily difficult to grasp the significance of the unexpected appearance. In biology there are always minor deviations from the expected. Most are probably quite unimportant and it would be an inconceivable waste of time to investigate them all. Amongst them, however, are the clues that lead to new discovery. Once the discovery has been made the clues are easy to recognise, but it is the mark of the first-rate research man that he can decide effectively which clue to follow and which to discard as an obvious red-herring.[1]

This is how Burnet described (forty-five years later) an event which occurred in 1923 and which was to serve as a vector, a giver-of-direction, to much of his scientific thought and work for the next two decades.

D'Herelle had assumed that there was just the one type, the bacteriophage. Burnet felt that there were probably many and proceeded to collect types from patients, from laboratory cultures, from the faeces of pigs, cows, horses, and chickens whenever he visited his brother's dairy farm. By immunological methods he showed that they were indeed different: he injected a rabbit with phage X, and the rabbit developed antibodies (in those days an antiserum) to phage X, which would kill phage X in the laboratory dish but would leave other phages unaffected. Unaffected phages could therefore be treated as phage Y and by a repeat of the technique, phage Z could be separated from phage Y, and so on until at least a dozen different groups of phage had been identified. For nearly twenty years there was a continuous strand of interest in phages and output of work on them in Burnet's scientific life story, but the peak of his interest in this subject came in the early 1930's, when he was studying a type of phage found in mouse typhoid bacilli. None of his techniques could rid his laboratory strain of these bacilli from their "disease," and they continued to produce small traces of phage; yet when the bacterial cells were broken open by a second type of phage specially introduced for the purpose, no trace of the continuously produced phage could be found. It prompted Burnet to propose that the infectious phage somehow combined with the genetic material of the bacteria and multiplied in step with its host until some outside environmental factor brought about a change in the situation. Then the phage suddenly started multiplying out of step with the bacteria and thus appeared as a true parasite in the host cells, visible to the outside world as an infectious disease.

A modern authority, Gunther Stent, writing in 1963 and quoted by Burnet, said that the work of Burnet and the Hungarian biochemist Schlesinger in the early 1930's

> foreshadowed the rise of bacterial genetics and molecular biology, disciplines that were to reach their heyday only twenty-five years later. . . . In 1936 Schlesinger's premature death ended his work and Burnet turned from bacteriophages to focus his attention on animal viruses. Since none of their collaborators or disciples continued this truly pioneering work in exact experimentation on bacterial viruses the continuity of modern phage work really dates from 1938 when Max Delbruck took up work in this field.[2]

Yet Burnet kept up at least a theoretical interest in the field, predicting in 1944 that "the study of micro-organismal genetics will show that bacterial hereditary mechanisms are accurately quantised and provide data of fundamental importance for the interpretation of organic evolution." And he was right.

But the Australian's main interest had indeed turned towards animal viruses, largely because he had spent two important years, 1932–33, working with the Medical Research Council virology team at Hampstead in London. He was not one of the small group that isolated the influenza virus for the first time by managing to infect ferrets with the disease, but he was near enough to them to be stopped on the stairs at Hampstead and told by a delighted Laidlaw, "The ferrets are sneezing." When he returned to his beloved Melbourne he concentrated on work on influenza for many years. Again, the details of this work are not directly germane to the development of his theories on immunology, but the techniques he worked out for studying influenza do have a direct bearing on the matter.

Burnet's chief technical achievement was the development of chick-embryo culture methods; in other words, he learned how to grow viruses in hen's eggs, following up the original discovery by the American Goodpasture. In 1935 and immediately thereafter, Burnet obtained influenza virus from nurses during a 'flu epidemic in the Melbourne Hospital Nurses' Home, transferred it to ferrets as a method of isolation, and then put drops of infected fluid onto the outer membranes of chicks growing inside their eggs. After about twenty passages from one egg to another, it became plain from spots and thickened patches on the membrane that the virus was adapting to growing on this medium. After another dozen transfers the spots were numerous. Burnet had achieved the technical success of adapting human influenza in at least one strain so that it would grow on chick-embryo membrane. The virus of influenza was available for study and for calculations on such matters as the amount of antibody present in human beings. Other scientists in many parts of the world followed Burnet's lead. Some of the subsequent discoveries were his own; some developments came from other people. By the end of the Second World War, when Burnet himself was working on the possibility of a live attenuated influenza vaccine, it had been discovered that the influenza virus as it adapted to growth on the egg membrane also became more virulent for chicks. Furthermore, it had been shown that the virus could also be grown on the body of the chick embryo itself and in the amniotic fluid immediately surrounding the embryo. Virus taken from the human being directly would also grow in the amniotic fluid, but it would not grow in the allantoic fluid—the outer "water-jacket" inside the egg—until it had been multiplying for at least two or three days in the amniotic fluid or inner "water-jacket." By these techniques and by immunological typing of the viruses grown in these ways, it was discovered that swine fever and fowl plague were caused by the same viruses that cause influenza in man. Influenza itself was shown to be caused by viruses of at least two major groups, the so-called A and B groups, which are antigenically different. Both would therefore have to be attenuated and used in any vaccine which could protect human beings against all 'flu.

By this time, 1945, Burnet had become acknowledged as one of the world leaders in the field of virology and immunology. He had been offered chairs and directorships in both the U.S.A. and Great Britain, he had given official lectures and been awarded medals in both countries. But he had also just accepted the directorship of the Walter and Eliza Hall Institute of Medical Research at Melbourne, the laboratory in which he had done most of his work. He was a determined Australian. In describing how he rejected an invitation to a full professorial chair at Harvard in 1945, he writes:

> In a curiously illogical fashion I have a deep emotional attachment to Australia, and I have never quite tolerated or forgotten the condescension of the English to colonials that was evident in pre-War days and is still not wholly dead. I have been treated with extraordinary generosity by the academic worlds of England and America but I am an Australian and through all my work there was a little extra drive which might be expressed in our own idiom "that I'd bloody well show them that we can do as well in this country as anywhere else." [3]

Later in his life this attitude, or something very like it, became an important theme in Burnet's work. He probably more than anyone else used his world influence to direct the attention and finances of his fellow countrymen towards scientific research, until today it is certainly true to say that

Australia is scientifically the most developed nation in the Southern Hemisphere.

But as well as this spiritual goad of a "scientific patriotism," there are other reasons why Burnet should have made the imaginative leaps that we call discoveries. As he said of himself, referring to his youth in the early years of this century, spent in country towns in the state of Victoria where his father was bank manager, "I am by temperament an ecologist, a naturalist, a collector of letters, a snapper-up of unconsidered trifles." There was no scientific strain in his family; there were also no scientists in those rural areas of Australia seventy years ago. He was simply a clever boy with no particular inclinations. But there was a strong strain of Scottish tradition and blood in his family and a Scottish belief in education. So he passed through the local state schools in Traralgon and Terang, to Geelong College and Melbourne University, with the intention of becoming a doctor. He was, on his own admission, a shy and rather lonely boy, and his consuming hobby was the collection of beetles, which he carried on to a stage which might be described as that of advanced amateur. From somewhere in this background arose what seems to me the crucial intellectual trait of the man—his habit of relating those phenomena which interested him to the general evolutionary background. Whether it was the intellectual isolation of a clever boy in a rural society or the close relation of a country boy to the teeming and exciting wildlife of Australia, or whether it was the actual study of beetles, is impossible to say. Certainly the result was that he attempted to find the evolutionary perspective in which he could place beetles, bacteriophage, virus, or the antibody that interested him.

When I met him in London briefly, in 1968, he had retired from academic and laboratory work. He was chairman of the Commonwealth Foundation, a charitable fund in the modern sense of that word, not receiving money donated by individuals and devoted to handing out soup to the hungry, but a fund to which the nations of the British Commonwealth contributed according to their wealth and from which useful projects of research and development were supported. Sir Macfarlane Burnet, comparatively slight of figure, gray-haired but still retaining a commanding quality in his blue eyes, still firm and clear in speech and idea, claimed to be still, at bottom, somewhat shy. My own impression was of enthusiasm rather than shyness, of drive rather than academic isolation. But the important point was that he claimed that he had found for the Commonwealth Foundation an "ecological niche," an area of human activity which was not overpopulated with rival organisations. This "niche," he said, was the area of medium-sized projects not requiring extremely advanced techniques. Typical of the work of the Foundation was the setting up of training schemes for laboratory and hospital technicians and nurses in East Africa—not large projects requiring massive governmental support or the latest scientific equipment, but considerably larger than private charitable schemes could consider. Working on the fringes of politics and government he had the same intellectual approach: the viewing of an operation in terms of the whole ecology, the organic evolution of the necessary services of modern life.

Burnet traces his own mental processes leading towards the discovery of immunological tolerance from his decision to write a semi-popular book, *The Biological Aspects of Infectious Diseases*. He began work on it about 1937 and published in 1940. The book was geared to "look at the whole process from a consistently ecological and evolutionary angle." It started from the question, "What happened when a primeval amoeba first discovered it could live by swallowing and digesting smaller microorganisms which were like itself single cells?" Somehow one organism must chemically disintegrate the other without damaging itself. And this seemed to lead to the necessity of some chemical definition of "self" and "not-self." (We have seen that early German immunologists like Loeb had considered this problem thirty years earlier.)

In the late 1930's the production of antibody was clearly understood as a major factor in the immune response, though there was nothing satisfactory in the way of a theory about how it was done. But in those years, diphtheria was just being overcome as a regular killer of thousands of children in Western countries, the Schick test was very much in the minds of most laboratory workers. This consisted of injecting a minute amount of diphtheria toxin under a child's skin. If the child has had a mild or non-lethal attack of diphtheria he will have been subjected to a certain amount of the toxin produced by the diphtheria bacilli (and in diphtheria, it is the toxin, a natural by-product of the bacillus, which causes the damage to human bodies). The child's body will have manufactured antibody to the toxin—an antitoxin—and in this case the Schick test will produce no outward signs, for the antitoxin will neutralise the toxin. A child who has not been immunised naturally against diphtheria toxin will show a red inflamed patch at the site of the injection, and will need to be vaccinated against the disease.

Work of this sort resulted in the knowledge that antibodies were produced not only against organisms, but against toxins and against bodies like the red blood cells of sheep and substances like egg white. It was known, furthermore, that antitoxin was a globulin molecule, one of the class of globulins found in all blood, and it was assumed that all antibodies were similarly globulins, which are protein molecules. Scientists learned as well that the antitoxin acted by uniting firmly with the toxin, and seemed to achieve its neutralising effect by smothering the toxin with itself and thus presenting a "self" surface to the rest of the body.

This in turn seemed to imply a "lock-and-key" relationship between antibody and antigen; an actual fitting together of two molecules. Since no antibody to diphtheria toxin could in those days be shown to exist in the body before either infection or immunisation, and since antitoxin could be shown in vast quantities after immunisation, it was reasonable to assume, as Burnet did in 1937, that in some way the antigen, the toxin, provided some sort of model, and the body built defensive antitoxin to fit the toxin in the lock-and-key manner. In modern terms Burnet then accepted an "instructive" theory, a theory that the antigen instructed the body, by its arrival and physical presence, as to the shape of the antibody that must be produced to neutralise it.

Burnet adopted two ideas in his book, which were to be of importance later. First, he believed that the "instruction" took place at the cellular level. This meant that the incoming antigen impressed its shape on a cell responsible for manufacturing antibody, rather than on antibody molecules themselves. Second, and more important, because more significant for the future, he introduced for the first time the notion that antibody-producing cells would have to be capable of producing daughter cells that could manufacture the same antibody as the parent.

Burnet admits in his autobiography, *Changing Patterns,* how far he still was from what we and he would now regard as the truth: "I assumed that the phagocytic cells conspicuous in spleen and lymph glands, the macrophages, were the antibody-producing cells. The lymphocyte, central to all modern discussion, was merely a cell of 'obscure function.'"

The situation remained static for nearly ten years. The immunologists and, indeed, nearly all the scientists were deeply involved in the war efforts of their various countries.

In the course of these efforts naturally there was a considerable build-up of scientifically established data on immune phenomena and antibody production—largely a by-product of the war work of producing vaccines for the armies. The instructive theories of antibody production held the theoretical stage and were supported by such great authorities as Linus Pauling, probably the most brilliant and original chemist America has ever produced. By the time everybody had sorted themselves out after the end of the war, "the study of immunology, quite apart from its practical importance, had accumulated a sufficiently large, ordered and consistent mass of facts to challenge chemists, biochemists, geneticists and others to carry their techniques into the field." The words are those of one of the standard textbooks on immunology, *Immunology for Students of Medicine* by Humphrey and White. The authors go on to say, "The time was also ripe for an attempt to assemble the facts into some general theoretical framework. Any hypothesis needed to explain not only how or why an immune response occurs following the introduction of foreign antigenic material, but also why there is no response to an animal's own bodily constituents which would be effective antigens in another species." [4]

Three sets of interesting facts emerged in the years 1946–49. First was Owens's discovery that twin calves, even when they are not identical twins, have in their blood streams red cells that are genetically the property of both individuals. This is basically because of a peculiarity in the placenta of the cow, which ensures that in the comparatively rare cases of twinning, the two calves share a single fused placenta. Thus their blood streams can mix before birth. Owens showed that in the case of two non-identical twin calves, red blood cells from Calf 1 could be found in Calf 2, and vice versa throughout their lives. Whereas in cases where the calves were not twins, injecting red cells from Calf 1 into Calf 2 was known certainly to cause Calf 2 to develop antibody and destroy the red cells from Calf 1. In other words, the twin calves were "tolerant" of each other's red blood cells.

The second line of thought came from Burnet's own particular work, the growth of influenza virus in chick embryos. Adult hens could certainly be infected with influenza virus and could develop antibodies to the virus. Yet chicks born from eggs in which the influenza virus had been grown in the allantoic fluid, where there had been millions of virus particles in the allantoic cavity, would grow up without antibody to influenza. Burnet himself checked this fact, using other antigens, such as red blood cells of sheep, and found again that the chick would grow up without antibodies to the introduced invader. It established the fact that there was a period of growth before which antibodies could not be formed.

Finally, there was the historic case of the disease of laboratory mice called LCM (lymphocytic chorio-meningitis). This disease caused Shope, a famous figure in the development of the cancer-virus stream of scientific thought and work, to become seriously ill at the Rockefeller Institute in 1937. Eventually it turned out that the LCM virus infected baby mice before they were born, and in these cases the mice lived on happily, producing no immune response to the virus and remaining unharmed by the continued presence and multiplication of the virus in their cells. If, however, the blood of one of these infected mice was transferred to the brain of another mouse of the same genetic stock, but uninfected from before birth, the recipient mouse would die of LCM.

In 1949, therefore, Burnet, with his Melbourne colleague Frank Fenner, published a monograph on the production of antibody suggesting that it should be possible to produce "tolerance" to an antigen artificially by injecting the animal with the antigen before it was born. For this suggestion he was awarded, jointly with Medawar, the Nobel prize in 1960. There are some nicely balanced gentle ironies about this. Burnet himself failed to prove his point experimentally—it was Medawar's work which settled the issue. But Burnet perfectly rightly holds that his suggestion about artificially produced immunological tolerance was but a stopping point on the way to his much more important theory of clonal selection as the basis of immune response—and for clonal selection he did not win a Nobel prize.

Burnet, of course, tried to show how to produce artificial tolerance experimentally, and it is interesting to see why he failed. He injected chick embryos with doses of influenza virus. He had been doing so for years and he knew that such chicks grew up normally without antibody to the virus. But this was not tolerance, for when he gave influenza virus to such chicks in adulthood they duly produced antibody in the normal way. Similar results followed with the use of other antigens, and these negative results were published. The point is that to produce tolerance the antigen must not only be presented to the embryo before antibody production can begin, but must continue to be present in the recipient system for the tolerance to hold into adult life. This can be expressed by saying that the deception must be continuous for it to continue to work.

For what seem to be purely historical reasons based on his own previous work, Medawar worked with skin grafts. In these cases, naturally, the antigen of the graft donor's cells is continuously present in the recipient system to keep up the deception—but more of that in the next chapter.

At this stage in the story it is necessary to insert two points. First, later work has shown that tolerance to foreign antigens can be induced in other ways than by prenatal injection—for instance, truly massive doses of antigen can induce tolerance in adult animals, presumably by swamping the defences, and this tolerance can be maintained by repeated applications of the antigen.

The second point refers back to the ideas of self and notself. Artificially induced tolerance by prenatal injection is essentially a matter of inducing the body to accept a foreign antigen as self by introducing it before the "self-determination" system is fully working. As long as that antigen remains in the system, the body will continue to regard it as self because it was "taught" to do so when the learning process was active. We do not know what the learning process is, but obviously it must be one of learning not to attack all those components found in the body at the time. It is quite possible that this learning is similar in nature to the swamping process which we assume produces tolerance in adulthood—that is to say, there is so much antigen that all the lymphocytes carrying the appropriate antibody are "taken out," to use a military phrase of the moment. Lymphocytes emerging at the start of the learning process which carried antibody to the body's own antigens might be similarly "mopped up" by the vast quantity of native antigen.

These two notes illustrate how significant Burnet's proposal was, although it was to lead to something even more important. The textbooks confirm this view in measured prose:

> Although the mechanism is still obscure and probably not as simple as Burnet and Fenner originally conceived it to be, the fulfilment of their prediction not only opened a new chapter of great potential importance in immunology, but it indicated that the biological phenomena of immunology could be fruitfully approached from a broad theoretical angle. This alone has provided a very powerful additional incentive to research on the fundamental nature of the immune response.[5]

In other words, the discovery of immunological tolerance was not only of importance in itself but also made immunology exciting again, exciting enough to attract some of the best brains in science.

But for Burnet it was "back to the egg," for it was from work on chick embryos that the next important point in the theory of immunology arose. Simonsen, a Dane, established a phenomenon which Medawar and his colleagues had missed in their earliest work, the phenomenon known as "graft-versus-host" reaction. A recipient animal normally rejects a graft by its immune responses, so the graft tissue will carry its donor's immune mechanism, or part of it, and the graft will try to reject the host by using its own immune response. Simonsen discovered this, not by using skin grafts but by injecting blood from a hen into a chick embryo through one of the embryo's veins, within the egg. He noted that large white nodules appeared in the spleen of the embryo. However, if he used blood from a hen of a very pure genetic strain, and injected it into an embryo of the same strain, the spleen did not contain any nodules. In fact, if the hen and the egg were so closely related genetically that the tissues of both carried the same antigens, the graft of blood did not attack the host embryo.

In Burnet's Melbourne laboratories the same thing was shown in a different way by one of his collaborators, the American Dr. Georgie Boyer (a lady whom Burnet describes as the most popular person ever to work at his institute). She showed that if hen blood cells were spread over the outer membrane of the chick embryo, the same membrane on which Burnet had started growing influenza virus, small white spots would appear. These spots were distinct enough to be counted. Burnet took over the technique from Boyer and it was in fact the final spell of work that he carried out with his own hands at the laboratory bench. He showed that the reaction was "graft-versus-host" reaction; he demonstrated further that the spots were caused by white blood cells from the hen; he further showed that the white cells proliferated at the site of the reaction—proliferation of cells was a vital part of the immune response.

The final link in the intellectual chain, according to Burnet himself, was the discovery by another Danish immunologist, Jerne, then working at Caltech, that a horse possessed measurable amounts of antibody to a bacteriophage before it was injected. Jerne therefore speculated that all animals had in their bodies small amounts of antibody specific to all antigens and that this natural antibody, when it met its appropriate antigen, combined with it. On being taken up by the phagocytic cells, it somehow then directed those cells to produce further quantities of antibody. This explained tolerance, but it did not fit with the growing body of knowledge of how protein was manufactured in the body (antibody is protein) and it did nothing to account for the presence of the natural antibody. Burnet met Jerne in 1955. He could not accept the Dane's theories, but was impressed by his data. Two years later, in 1957, he produced the basis of what is now accepted as the clonal theory in a famous paper entitled "A Modification of Jerne's Theory of Antibody Production Using the Concept of Clonal Selection." It was published in the Australian *Journal of Science*.

The essence of the theory is that at some stage of embryonic development there must be an extraordinary diversification or "randomisation" of that part of the genetic code which specifies the apparatus for the production of antibody. This diversification is so enormous that a coding for the production of every possible type of antibody is generated. Once a coding for a particular antibody is completed, the cells containing that coding are fixed and all subsequent descendants of those few cells are clonally derived.[6] This means that they are produced by splitting of the cell. Consequently, the genetic material, including the coding for that particular antibody, remains unchanged and all descendants of those cells will produce just that one antibody.

Burnet stated that an essential part of his theory was that these clonally derived, "expendable" body cells (now known to be the lymphocytes) must carry on their surface an example of the antibody they are coded to produce. The arrival of antigen stimulates the proliferation of those cells carrying fitting antibody. Since these cells proliferate while other similar cells carrying non-fitting antibody do not multiply at that moment of arrival of the antigen, the cells with the fitting antibody are "selected" in the Darwinian sense.

The predictions in this original paper included the idea that some of the proliferating "selected" cells would develop into forms capable of producing quantities of specific antibody. Thus eventually the blood serum would be seen to contain large amounts of antibody, even to the extent of becoming briefly the "antiserum" of the traditional clinical immunologist. Others of the descendants of the selected cells would simply be reproductions of the parent cells and so an increased number of these cells would be available to mount the rapid counter-attack which we observe as immunity.

As the title of the paper suggests, it was simply an account of a method of antibody production to meet specific antigens. But manifestly such an account fits into the broader theory of self and not-self. And it is now the widely accepted theory which forms the base of immunology.

As to the publication of such an important theory in the comparative obscurity of the Australian *Journal of Science*, Burnet admits in his autobiography that this was a combination of national pride and a desire to "have his cake and eat it." If wrong, the theory would not have been widely read in Europe and America; if right, he had established scientific priority of publication for Australia.

Two months after the publication in September 1957, Joshua Lederberg visited Burnet in Melbourne, officially to see the latest work on influenza virus. The meeting instead developed into providing the first proof of part of the clonal theory. Using Lederberg's techniques for isolating single cells, he and Burnet's chief assistant, Gus Nossal, took cells from the lymph glands of rats that had been inoculated with two types of bacteria. If single cells could only produce one type of antibody, as the clonal theory proposed, then the antibody from these single lymph gland cells ought to kill only one of the two types of bacteria with which the rats had been inoculated. In a few days Nossal and Lederberg proved that this was the case—a cell which produced antibody to kill bacteria X could not produce antibody to kill bacteria Y. The "instructive" theories of antibody production were dead and the clonal theory was launched.

It took ten years for the theory to gain anything like world-wide acceptance. If any one field of study can be considered to have proved the clonal theory, it has been the study of Bence-Jones proteins excreted by patients suffering from the type of cancer known as myeloma. This is now interpreted as a cancer caused by a single clone of immunological cells "running wild" and producing enormous quantities of antibodies or the "chains" of antibodies; all these antibody molecules turn out to be specific for only one antigen in any particular case.

At the Cold Spring Harbor Symposium of 1967 it was finally accepted—not of course by motion carried by vote—that the work of the previous five years or so, including that on myeloma proteins, had pretty well established the clonal selection theory. It had of course been modified in detail over the years, having endured a rough passage through to scientific acceptance. In Burnet's words, the essence of it could now be expressed in five points:

1. Antibody is produced by cells, to a pattern which is laid down by the genetic mechanism in the nucleus of the cell.

2. Antigen has only one function, to stimulate cells capable of producing the kind of antibody which will react with it, to proliferate and liberate their characteristic antibody.

3. Except under quite abnormal conditions one cell produces only one type of antibody.

4. All descendants of an antibody-producing cell produce the same type of antibody.

5. There is a genetic mechanism capable of generating in random fashion a wide but not infinite range of patterns so that there will be at least some cells that can react with any foreign material that enters the body.[7]

For those who, like myself, tend to be irritated when dramatists or novelists seem to impose a form on the randomness of life, there is an even more exacerbating lesson to be drawn from the history of Sir Frank Macfarlane Burnet's progress to the idea of clonal selection theory. At the Cold Spring Harbor Symposium, the man who gave the final summary congratulating Burnet on "the vindication of his clonal selection theory of acquired immunity," was Jerne. And the man who initially supported him in his theory and provided the first experimental evidence once it had been published, Joshua Lederberg, was the supreme bacterial geneticist.

Chapter 6

The Beginning of Modern Immunology

The value of a scientific theory lies not in its approach to absolute truth, which we can never know, but in the generation of experiments designed to refute or confirm it, experiments which themselves produce new knowledge. (This is my own gloss on Sir Karl Popper's theories of scientific progress.)

The value of Sir Macfarlane Burnet's propositions about immunological tolerance lies at least in one respect in the stimulation they gave to Sir Peter Medawar to provide experimental proof of the theory. And the value of Medawar's work in London in the early 1950's lies not only in the proof of the theory of tolerance but also in the excitement it engendered among many scientists, in the intellectual boost it gave to immunology, and in the fact that it suddenly made the concept of transplant surgery feasible.

Yet it was a curious set of chance circumstances that brought Medawar into this field, and these circumstances emphasise the point about the situation of immunology at the end of the Second World War. Medawar was basically a zoologist, who had started research work at the Sir William Dunn School of Pathology in Oxford—the same establishment that housed Gowans when much later he elucidated the role of the lymphocyte. During the war, Medawar had been asked by the Medical Research Council to work on the problem of the inability to graft skin from one person to another, a problem which was of considerable importance in the many cases of Air Force fighter pilots badly burned when their planes were shot down. Just after the end of the war, back at Oxford, Medawar had been feeling very uncertain about the direction his research should take and in 1946 he was actually offered a position in Melbourne by Macfarlane Burnet. Instead, after a couple of years as professor at Birmingham University, he moved to the chair of Zoology at University College, London.

Medawar, like Burnet, had been interested by Owens's University of Wisconsin work on cattle twins. Following up his own war-time work, he tried grafting skin between such cattle twins and found that, despite the plainly demonstrable genetic differences between the two calves, they would accept skin grafts from each other. Up to this time successful grafts had been confined to those between identical twins, where the two animals have sprung from a single fertilised egg and are genetically and antigenically the same. (Grafts of the cornea of the eye, where there is no blood supply, and therefore neither circulating lymphocytes nor antibody, had been performed as long ago as 1852.) But these calf-grafting experiments, which were done with Rupert Billingham as Medawar's assistant, led nowhere in particular. Meanwhile Burnet's proposals about immune tolerance had been published in 1949.

So, by drawing on his own work, and taking some leads from the published work of Owens and Lilley, who had followed up Owens's finding on calves, Medawar conceived the project of a definite program of work to test the Burnet hypothesis. In 1951 a young zoology student from Medawar's old department at Birmingham, Lindsay Brent, came to join Billingham to complete the team of three; the work on tolerance was to be Brent's Ph.D. thesis. (He is now professor of immunology at St. Mary's Hospital in London; Billingham holds a professorship in the United States.)

Medawar's plan was to take mice of highly inbred strains, to inject the embryos of one strain with cells of another strain taken from adults, and then to test by skin grafting whether tolerance of the second strain had been achieved. There was one important technical achievement, not his own, which laid the foundation of his experimental techniques. This was the development of extremely pure strains of inbred laboratory mice. By repeated mating of brothers with sisters and by back-crossing offspring with parents it had proved possible to produce strains of mice in which every individual was almost completely genetically identical with every other individual. It is almost as though they were all identical twins, or—to put it another way—the genetic variation which is the chief feature of sexual reproduction is so reduced that one generation of creatures is almost as like its parents as in clonal or vegetative reproduction. Complete genetic similarity is not achieved in these pure strains, but at least as far as the antigens on the surface of their body cells are concerned they appear to be almost identical one with another, though it is now known there is one qualification to this.

The team at University College used two of these pure strains of mice—"Strong A," which are white, and "CBA," which are brown mice. Both strains of animals are still being used today in zoology and genetics laboratories, but their importance to Medawar lay not only in their viability but also in the extremely strong mutual rejection reactions. These reactions were so definite that it was perfectly possible to measure the time taken to reject a graft in days and so provide a quantitative system of measuring the strength of rejection. Thus an untreated A-strain mouse would normally reject a graft of skin from CBA in ten or eleven days. If, however, the A strain mouse had previously been immunised against the CBA strain by injections of cells from CBA mice, then the rejection of the skin graft would be much more rapid, taking only five or six days. This "second set" response is exactly the same as the immunity against infectious disease provided by having suffered a previous attack by the disease. (Referring back to the qualification of complete genetic identity mentioned in the previous paragraph, much later it was discovered that males of these strains carried an extremely weak antigen which was not shared by females; it is the weakest antigen that has yet been found, but by itself it can cause rejection of a graft after sixty or one hundred days.)

The technique adopted by the team in the early days was to open the abdomen of a pregnant mouse and find the womb, which is transparent in mice. Through the wall of the womb they would then inject doses of cells from adult CBA mice into 15- to 18-day-old embryos of A strain mice; and of course repeat the operation, putting adult A strain cells into CBA embryos. Two or three days later the litter would be born, since the gestation period of a mouse is twenty days. When the young were five or six weeks old, they would receive a skin graft from adult animals of the strain whose cells had been injected into them prenatally. At the same time, control experiments on untreated mice established the normal pattern of rejection.

Billingham and Medawar had perfected the grafting operation in the early days of the project in 1951. This consisted of carefully preparing a bed in the skin of the animal due to receive the graft, and then cutting an exactly matching piece of skin from the donor. After the graft had been made, a thin plaster was placed over the spot and left there for ten days. On the tenth day the plaster was taken off and it was then a matter simply of observing the progress of the graft. There might be inflammation and the sloughing off of the received piece of skin if rejection was normal. Acceptance of the graft would be signified by the growth of its natural hair on the transferred piece of skin, so that tolerance was signified by patches of white hair on brown mice or brown hair on white mice.

The picture of work here is very different from the activities of Burnet in Australia. He was already a world-recognised figure on account of his work on virus and bacteriophage before he produced theories on tolerance and clonal selection. He was the director of a modern research institute. The three men at University College had two small laboratories occupied by Medawar and Brent, the professor and the research student, respectively, while Billingham worked in the largest of their three rooms. The building in which they worked was old and old-fashioned. And though the conditions were by no means slummy or overcrowded, with Great Britain's financial state in the early 1950's Medawar had to scheme to get extra grants from funds in the United States for major pieces of equipment like an ultra-centrifuge and to support the rather expensive mouse colonies they needed. There was also a great deal of highly skilled clinical operative manipulation in the skin grafting and in the injections into embryos. Usually two of the three men would be working together on opposite sides of a laboratory bench as they handled their mice, but these pairs would change into every possible permutation of two out of three.

During these long, boring, and repetitive operations there was much conversation, and since Medawar is a highly civilised and cultivated man, with deep interests in philosophy and music, it is easy to understand why Brent, for instance, remembers this as the most highly educative period of his

life. (I have found personally that meeting Sir Peter Medawar usually leaves me a great deal wiser, often about problems of which I had previously been totally ignorant.)

However, early in 1951 for a spell of about six months
there were very few results to show for all this work. They
did not know which cells or how many to inject into the embryos. They lost many litters altogether. There were undoubtedly times of depression when they wondered if there
was such a phenomenon as artificial tolerance at all or
whether their methods were totally wrong. But there were
just enough results to encourage them to persevere, and for
nine months in 1952 they worked very hard indeed. They
changed this part of their technique and that. They gave up
opening the abdomens of the pregnant mice; instead, as their
skill in manipulation grew with practice, they were able simply to make an incision through the skin. They then injected
the tolerance-producing adult cells into the embryos through
the stomach wall and the uterus wall in one go. This was less
efficient but obviously better for the animals and it reduced
the number of litters lost.

By the end of 1952 they were getting regular and encouraging results. Excitement began to grow. There was certainly
some phenomenon here among the white tufts of hair on
brown mice, a phenomenon which could be produced fairly
consistently by their techniques. Now this must be analysed
to decide what was really happening.

The first question to be asked was the immunologist's
question, Is this phenomenon specific? (They would probably have lost interest in the whole project if it had turned
out to be non-specific.) So they took the animals with the
biggest, best, most accepted, and hairiest grafts and gave
them skin grafts from a third pure strain of inbred mice.
They took, say, a CBA mouse, which their treatment by prenatal injection had made tolerant to the antigens of A strain

mice and which bore a prominent white patch of A strain hair to mark where it had accepted the A strain graft. And they grafted onto the other side of its chest a piece of skin from a third strain of mice, actually called "AU" mice. All AU skin grafts were rejected in precisely the normal time an untreated mouse needs to reject a graft from any other strain. So the tolerance they had produced was specifically a tolerance to the antigens of A strain mice. Repeat experiments showed that the A strain mice had likewise been made specifically tolerant to CBA antigens. Immunological tolerance is therefore a specific phenomenon. This was vitally important for enormous quantities of later work in this field.

Next, they wished to show whether this artificially induced tolerance was a generalised defect in the antibody-producing system of the treated mice or whether it was an inability to mount a specific immunological response. So they took a selection of untreated CBA mice and split them into two groups. One group was then injected with A strain cells and therefore immunised against A strain antigens. From these two groups they took lymph gland cells, and injected these cells into CBA mice which had been made tolerant to A strain cells and which bore healthy skin grafts from A strain mice. All the previously tolerant mice rejected their skin grafts, but those given the presensitised cells rejected their grafts more quickly than those given cells which had never previously encountered A strain antigens. This showed that tolerance is a defect in the capacity to produce a specific immune response.

It also partly answered such questions as, Has the resident graft been changed by its very residence? and Have the antigens of the resident graft been changed enough by residence to account for tolerance? Final rejection of this possibility came from a further series of experiments. Second grafts of skin onto tolerant animals showed that they were still tolerant. Then Medawar's team took healthy grafts and transferred them to untreated animals of both the donor and recipient strains: the animals of the donor strain accepted the skin from their own strains, but untreated animals of the recipient strain would not accept grafts which had been successful on their genetically equivalent relatives who had been rendered tolerant. Therefore the tolerance was not a change in the graft.

Finally, the results were confirmed by work with chick embryos, proving that the phenomenon was not restricted to mice. The work on chick embryos was stimulated by the example of the Czech immunologist Hashek, and consisted of fusing two chick embryos at the eleventh day of incubation (leaving nine days to full term) in such a way that the prenatal blood streams were mixed. Several pairs of chicks were successfully hatched and it was shown that, like twin calves, they were "chimaeras" with red cells from both individuals in both their blood streams. Later skin grafts between these pairs of chicks were successful.

The existence of artificially induced immunological tolerance was first published in a paper in *Nature*, the leading British scientific journal, in 1953. The full details of the work, confirming Burnet's predictions of 1949, appeared three years later (1956) in the *Royal Society Philosophical Transactions*, an appearance which was in itself an honor, for the Royal Society is the oldest scientific society in the world.

Before that, in 1955, Billingham and Brent had discovered that the period during which tolerance could be induced was not confined to the embryonic stage of development but extended to at least the first day or so after birth in the case of mice. In other words, the development of the self-recognition system and the ability to challenge not-self was certainly not completed at birth. In man it may be several months after birth before the system is fully operational.

From the point of view of technique, this discovery considerably simplified matters, for instead of the delicate probing of the pregnant mouse and the blind injection of cells into unseen embryos in the womb, it was now possible to produce tolerance by the injection of cells into the veins of perfectly visible and easily manipulated newborn mice within the first twenty-four hours of their life.

In some sense the proof of the existence of immunological tolerance and the demonstration that it could be artificially induced had most significance in terms of effects on the psychological and imaginative progress of immunology. It showed that immunology was the science of self in a new and more easily acceptable way: not only was the body defending itself against not-self bacteria; much more precisely, an individual, albeit a mouse, was defending itself against material from another individual. And the very method by which the defences could be breached, the method of deception if you like, emphasised that it was a matter of persuading one individual that another specific individual was self—as still other individuals could still be correctly recognised as not-self. Although there was no discovery of anything like a "self-marker flag," and there may never turn out to be such a thing, obviously the whole process was some sort of differentiation between self and not-self. And it was further obvious that this machinery of differentiation was a system that only became fully operational at some precise time in the individual's development—a measurable, discoverable system.

It seems to have been simply the historical accident of Medawar's previous involvement in problems of skin grafting that led him to choose this technique for looking into the question of the existence, or no, of immunological tolerance. It was therefore, in a sense, luck that enabled the English team to avoid the mistake made by Burnet, because the technical system they had chosen implied that the foreign antigens were continuously present in the recipient's system—this continuous presence of the foreign antigen being essential for keeping the tolerance in existence. But there can be little doubt that this was one of those scientific discoveries which, had it not been made by Medawar then, would undoubtedly have been made by someone else not long afterwards.

A time scale that may well have been changed by the fortuitous choice of skin grafts to demonstrate tolerance is that of transplant surgery. The possibility of organ transplants becoming a normal and regular feature of clinical treatment of disease was implicit in the new turn taken by immunology when Burnet began his theorising. However, only the fact that the new immunology was experimentally founded on transplantation accounts for transplantation becoming one of the major objectives of the new immunology. This rather curious development is emphasised by the fact that artificially induced tolerance is not yet the chosen method for persuading a patient's body to accept a graft from another individual—we make grafts acceptable by suppressing the production of specific antibody after a specific not-self has been recognised. (More details about this follow in Chapter 8.)

Medawar himself made this point to me in a BBC Third Programme broadcast in 1966. He had been awarded the Nobel Prize, jointly with Burnet, for his work in 1960, and he said:

> In reality I think I was awarded the Nobel prize for having studied the biological theory—the transplantation of tissues—and put it upon a sound experimental basis. The particular discovery was finding out that it is, in principle, possible to overcome the barrier that normally prevents the transplantation of tissues between different individuals. This barrier is an immunological barrier, and at the time we started it was

very far from obvious that this barrier could be broken down or that it would ever be possible to transplant tissues from one human being to another. We showed that it is possible— and in fact it is now possible by all kinds of different methods, not merely the one that we originally devised.[1]

In his autobiography Burnet tells of frequent meetings with Medawar in the 1950's, meetings that very often seemed to take place over beer and cheese in a London pub. It is a fascinating exercise of the imagination to try to recreate these encounters—the short, spare, erect Burnet, still a flavour of Scottish Presbyterian ancestry mingled with the slight but ever-present bristle of Australian national pride; and the tall, even-tempered, superbly civilised Medawar, Brazilian born of a Lebanese Arab trader looking back to the ancient Phoenician sea-traders as his ancestors, but who had been educated at a British public school and the University of Oxford.

In the BBC programme mentioned above I talked with Medawar about the nature of a new thought:

This is the creative or inspirational act, the nature of which is unknown. All one knows about it is that whatever precedes the entry of an idea into the mind is not known consciously. It is something subconscious. There is a piecing-together and putting-together of something in the mind, but unfortunately of this process nothing is known. There have been attempts to analyse the process. Coleridge, for example, believed that the creative process was a sort of microcosmic reproduction of the original Divine Creation. That really out of a formless chaos of words or vaguely formulated ideas, poetic ideas arose spontaneously in his mind. Now it happens that Coleridge has been the subject of a very great deal of critical and exegetic attention and it is more certainly true of Coleridge than of any other known man that his conception of the creative process was not correct; because almost all of his ideas can be traced back to something he read in the past, ideas known to have entered his mind. He put them together in a distinctive way, but they were not "original" in the sense that he used the word original—arising as it were out of chaos, out of nothing.

It is this type of thinking and interest, spreading so far beyond the experimental proof of immunological tolerance, that has made Medawar the leading scientist-advocate of a revolution in thinking about science and asking how it is actually done. This began with Sir Karl Popper, a philosopher by profession and a professor at the London School of Economics for much of his working life. This chapter opened with my gloss on Popper's theories. Now, to put the record straight, here are some of his own words, taken from the preface to his book *Conjectures and Refutations:*

> The way in which knowledge progresses, and especially our scientific knowledge, is by unjustified (and unjustifiable) anticipations, by guesses, by tentative solutions to our problems, by *conjectures*. These conjectures are controlled by criticism; that is by attempted *refutations*, which include severely critical tests. They may survive these tests; but they can never be positively justified: they can neither be established as certainly true nor even as probable (in the sense of the probability calculus). Criticism of our conjectures is of decisive importance: by bringing out our mistakes it makes us understand the difficulties of the problem which we are trying to solve. This is how we become better acquainted with our problem, and able to propose more mature solutions: the very refutation of a theory—that is, of any serious tentative solution to our problem—is always a step forward that takes us nearer to the truth. And this is how we can learn from our mistakes. . . .
>
> Those among our theories which turn out to be highly resistant to criticism, and which appear to us at a certain moment of time to be better approximations to truth than other known theories, may be described, together with reports of

their tests, as "the science" of that time. Since none of them can be positively justified, it is essentially their critical and progressive character—the fact that we can argue about their claim to solve our problems better than their competitors— which constitutes the rationality of science.[2]

To me this explanation comes nearest to what I have seen actually happening in science. Therefore I must plead guilty to inconsistency in having written that Medawar provided experimental proof of the truth of the idea of immunological tolerance. In extenuation, I quote the admission by Medawar, who published an article entitled "Is the Scientific Paper a Fraud?", that he has never printed a paper written in completely Popperian style. One can easily see that Medawar, whose main scientific work has been the checking and testing of a highly "improbable" hypothesis, would be attracted to Popper's ideas; in fact, he has turned into a great advocate of them.

Medawar delivered the Jayne Lectures for 1968 to the American Philosophical Society at the University of Pennsylvania, Philadelphia—since published as *Induction and Intuition in Scientific Thought*. In them Medawar argues that for the past hundred years the English-speaking world has been dominated by the opinion that scientific thinking is inductive, that the scientist argues from the particular to the general, collecting facts, perceiving among the facts some general law, making predictions about further facts from that law, then proving the law by experimentally checking the predictions. Mathematics, however, is deductive, arguing from a general axiom down to particular results. Then he points out (as Popper has done too) that as long ago as the seventeenth century the English philosopher Locke had shown that induction can never be a logically rigorous process. But, in any case, the theory is simply not supported by what goes on in practice:

Deductivism in mathematical literature and inductivism in scientific papers are simply the postures we choose to be seen in when the curtain goes up and the public sees us. The theatrical illusion is shattered if we ask what goes on behind the scenes. In real life discovery and justification are almost always different processes and a sound methodology must make it clear that they are so. . . .

[And a little later on] . . . Methodologists who have no personal experience of scientific research have been gravely handicapped by their failure to realise that nearly all scientific research leads nowhere—or if it does lead somewhere then not in the direction it started off with. In retrospect we tend to forget errors, so that the Scientific Method appears very much more powerful than it really is. . . . I reckon that for all the use it has been to science about four-fifths of my time has been wasted.[3]

Medawar finally plumps for what he calls the "hypo-thetico-deductive system" of explaining what actually happens in science, and this is essentially the explanation put forward by Popper. Medawar describes it with his inside experience:

Science in its forward motion is not logically propelled. Scientific reasoning is an exploratory dialogue that can always be resolved into two voices or two episodes of thought, imaginative and critical, which alternate and interact. In the imaginative episode we form an opinion, take a view, make an informed guess, which might explain the phenomena under investigation. The generative act is the formation of a hypothesis. . . . The process by which we come to formulate a hypothesis is not illogical, but non-logical, i.e. outside logic. But once we have formed an opinion we can expose it to criticism usually by experimentation; this episode lies within and makes use of logic, for it is an empirical testing of the logical consequences of our beliefs. . . . If our predictions are borne out then we are justified in extending a certain confidence to the hypothesis. If not, there must be something wrong, perhaps so wrong as to oblige us to abandon our hypothesis altogether.[4]

And he goes on to elaborate, in terms obviously drawn from his own experience in the laboratory, an implication of Popper's theories, that it is the "improbable" (in the mathematical sense) hypothesis that is most valuable. Medawar says that it is the risky, daring hypothesis, the hypothesis that might so easily not be true (remember Burnet publishing his clonal theory in the comparative obscurity of the Australian journal) that gives us special confidence when it stands up to the critical examination of experiment. This sort of approach accounts for so many of the human factors which are plainly visible in the scientific world. It allows for the drive and incentive of the individual in science, it provides for the factors of error and luck, and it also allows for the slow disappearance of a once-attractive theory. This again we know is what really happens to scientific theories, rather than their sudden execution by the rigorous logic implied in the traditional inductivist view of the demise of a theory.

Illustrating even more directly from his own experience —and this is also a significant point in the history of immunology—Medawar describes how he and his colleagues missed the clear evidence of "graft-versus-host" reaction which is now known to have been present in his early experiments. Although the facts were staring them in the face, they missed them because "they did not enter into our conception of what might be true or alternatively because of a mistaken belief that they could not be true." The "hypothetico" part of "hypothetico-deductive" is "the invention of a fragment of a possible world"—and this enters all scientific thinking, not just the great discoveries.

This view of the nature of scientific progress seems to me to be illustrated again and again in the story of immunology. But it is not a widely shared view. Particularly, it is not widely held in America. For instance, Burnet in his autobiographical description of his development of clonal selection theory writes:

> I have already said that I believe my most important contribution to science was the concept of clonal selection as applied to immunological theory. I think it is also correct to say that most American immunologists would take the point of view that although the modern approach to immunology has virtually all the features I described in 1957–59, my theoretical approach was almost irrelevant to the development of immunology. In their view the present position results simply from the accumulation of experimental data and has not been significantly influenced by my theoretical approach. I have much sympathy with this point of view, but for very ordinary human reasons I shall take the point of view that the whole philosophy of clonal selection amongst the somatic cells of the body was basically new, that it is very important for the understanding of human disease, and that a large number of immunologists and pathologists are still failing to understand it.[5]

In his final summing up Burnet returns to this theme, saying:

> I have been a fairly controversial figure in medical science and, as I may have indicated between the lines, there has been more than a sprinkling of sound and distinguished scientists who at one time or other have felt that I have been lacking in the first requirement of a scientist—that he should never move beyond what he can establish experimentally. It is probably more correct to put that point of view in the form that in any account of new experimental work, speculation should not appear; its proper place is elsewhere. I have broken

that rule too often, and, if anything, I have become worse as I got older.[6]

But he remains manifestly unrepentant.

In view of all this it is fascinating to read the remarks of one of the United States' most outstanding immunologists (many would say *the* greatest American immunologist), Professor Robert Good, giving the presidential address to the Sixtieth Annual Meeting of the American Society for Clinical Investigation (Atlantic City, May 1968), and describing his position in terms of the animal behaviourists: "A leader selected by previous vigor and successful defense of intellectual territories is placed in a central position, given an impossible task, and then dismissed from the group along with the aged cohorts. . . ." Good dealt with the nature of scientific progress and quoted Medawar and above all Popper with high approval. And in 1969, at a conference on tumours of invertebrates, Good gave a paper, now published as a monograph of the National Cancer Institute, which ended with the words:

> Our position is highly speculative. Its corollaries however present numerous working hypotheses which can be disproved and are thus of scientific merit. One of the most proximal of these corollaries is that malignancies either do not occur or occur only rarely among the invertebrates. It is with this hypothesis that we would like to challenge this symposium. A delightful achievement of this conference would be to prove us wrong and to establish that invertebrates do, indeed, have malignancies which occur with the frequency and variety so readily observed among all the vertebrates.[7]

I have not yet heard of any successful refutation of this conjecture.

Chapter 7

The Development
of the Science

Robert A. Good, Regents' Professor of Pediatrics and Microbiology at the Medical School of the University of Minnesota
in Minneapolis, is an extremely important figure in the story
of immunology. He is so for three reasons: firstly, for his own
discoveries; secondly, because his work represents both the
clinical approach and the detailed working-out of the mechanisms of the immune system; and thirdly, because he represents the American "style" and line of thought in the development of the science of self.

He is a Middle Westerner. Born in Minnesota, schooled
in Minneapolis, almost the whole of his working life, except
for a couple of years at the Rockefeller Institute for Medical
Research in New York, has been spent at the University of
Minnesota. To European eyes, at least, he is the very epitome
of the successful American academic. He works in a rich university, he controls a huge department, his students flow out
into the world of American research to become professors
and assistant professors themselves. His output, in terms of
scientific papers, is enormous—year after year after year the
Index Medicus lists between fifteen and twenty major papers
bearing his name, and the names of three, four, or five of his

colleagues and students. There is no hint here of three men working in dingy, elderly buildings in an unfashionable part of town, with the senior having to negotiate grants for an extra piece of equipment. Nor of a pugnacious Australian trying to persuade the world that a good idea might come out of Melbourne while simultaneously trying to persuade Melbourne that science is worthwhile. A typical paper by Robert Good is addressed from the Pediatric Research Laboratories of the Variety Club Heart Hospital and the Department of Microbiology of the University of Minnesota. It acknowledges grants from the U.S. Public Health Service, from the American Heart Association, the National Foundation, the American Cancer Society, the Minnesota Heart Association, and the Minnesota Chapter of the Arthritis Foundation. Add to this the fact that the University of Minnesota Medical School is closely linked with the world-famous Mayo Clinics at Rochester, and you have a man working in the American "style," at the apex of the highest reaches of American medicine, using the wealth and technical power of American society and culture, partaking of that particular energy which is typically American, to solve problems posed in different ways, with different working methods by scientists in other countries. And, since we have seen that he accepts a great deal of what Popper has to say, Good is also able to pose his own questions to his immunological colleagues around the world.

Good started as a brilliant medical student in the early 1940's. He became interested in immunology as a result of his first research project, though it was essentially a study of brain disease in rabbits caused by the herpes simplex virus— the virus that causes cold sores on human lips. By 1943 he was assisting Fred Kolouch in his work on plasma cells, and the significance here is that Kolouch was the man whose work started the trail that led to the discovery (by Astrid Fagraeus, a Swedish research worker) that the producers of antibody are the plasma cells. The discovery was made in 1946, and not only did it have its own importance, but it also finally pushed the phagocytes into a minor role in immune responses. The phagocytes had been steadily declining in interest since the palmy days of Metchnikoff and Almroth Wright. But until Fagraeus's definitive work (supported by parallel experiments by Coons) most people had been inclined to think, in the absence of a better alternative, that the phagocytes were somehow responsible for turning out antibody after they had ingested the combination of antigen and antibody. After 1946 it became clear that the plasma cells—which were found in lymphoid tissue, and which had been shown by Kolouch to proliferate wildly when the system was stimulated by antigen—were giant factories for the synthesis of protein, and that their output was gammaglobulin antibodies. (Not until much more recently did evidence begin to accumulate that the plasma cells are descendants of lymphocytes; this is hardly surprising since the lymphocyte consists of little more than a nucleus, whereas the cytoplasm, which is the area in which protein is synthesised, completely overshadows the nucleus in a plasma cell.)

This work of Good's with Kolouch was done when he was still a student. Shortly after getting his Ph.D. in 1947, he spent a couple of years at the Rockefeller Institute. While there, Good became involved in another of the main streams of immunological development, the examination of the myeloma proteins—a line of progress which did much to establish the clonal selection theory on a firm basis of fact.

It seems that work derived essentially from a clinical basis, that is, from a study of human patients and in attempts to relieve and cure them, has always been the main attraction for Robert Good. Back in Minnesota from 1950 onwards he returned to his specialisation in pediatrics, the diseases and problems of children. After showing particular interest in rheumatic fever, the real excitement began with a study of cases of agammaglobulinaemia: a grave deficiency in gammaglobulins, and hence in antibodies, resulting in poor response to infection. It is quite correct to describe agammaglobulinaemia as a rare disease of children. (In the even rarer cases of adults suffering from lack of gammaglobulins, it is strictly "acquired" agammaglobulinaemia.) This conjures up the picture of a rather "ivory tower" medical man specialising in one very uncommon disease. But the disease is rare and confined to children simply because the body is so defenceless against invasion that the patient usually dies of an overwhelming infection by some quite common bacteria, virus, or fungus. The essential nature of the disease is simple and quite basic to survival. It is obviously an immunological disease, a deficiency in the immunological system. And it is because his basic interest is in clinical diseases of the immunological system, and because these diseases are furthermore usually confined to children (it being difficult for the patient ever to reach adulthood), that Good is a professor of pediatrics by official title, although he is by repute one of the world's greatest immunologists.

This brings into focus the central point of Good's philosophy, namely, that diseases are "experiments of Nature," which can be interpreted by the scientist to produce results just as valuable as those obtained from the interpretation of experiments performed in the laboratory. He made this abundantly clear in his presidential address to the American Society for Clinical Investigation in 1967. "I intend to argue," he said then, "that the experiments performed by Nature, especially in our clinics and hospitals, have represented historically, and continue to represent, an extraordinary resource for scientific endeavor." And he went on to quote a letter written in London in 1657 by William Harvey, the discoverer of the circulation of the blood:

Learned Sir . . . It is even so. Nature is nowhere accustomed more openly to display her secret mysteries than in cases where she shows traces of her workings apart from the beaten path; nor is there any better way to advance the proper practice of medicine than to give our minds to the discovery of the usual law of Nature, by the careful investigation of cases of rarer forms of disease. For it has been found in almost all things that what they contain of useful or of applicable, is hardly perceived unless we are deprived of them, or they become deranged in some way. . . .

Later in the same address Good explains why he finds these "experiments of Nature" such a valuable source of inspiration: "Not the least responsible for the effectiveness of Nature's experiments is their power to motivate the physicians and the scientists involved. Certainly an important share of science's great debt to medicine is traceable to the natural human motive to alleviate suffering and the natural desire to treat and prevent disease." [1]

Agammaglobulinaemia (the disease of being unable to manufacture gammaglobulin and therefore antibodies) can be regarded as a natural experiment, and the scientific study of patients with this disease should show how they differ from normal people in other ways. Hence it should be possible to establish the mechanisms by which gammaglobulins and antibodies are made in normal people. It was precisely by studying such cases that Good made his first important discovery: that plasma cells, which we know are the producers of antibodies, could not be found in any of the tissues of the body where blood is normally formed. And, further, that sufferers from agammaglobulinaemia could not be persuaded to develop any plasma cells even when they were extensively stimulated with antigens which in normal people cause plasma cells to appear in large numbers—and, of course, produce antibody in large quantities.

Apart from the bone marrow, which is one of the chief

sources of cells in blood formation, and the other blood-forming tissues (technically the reticulo-endothelial system), plasma cells are most usually found in the lymphoid tissue. Studying this part of the system in agammaglobulin-aemia patients led Good to notice that there were different types of tissue in such areas as the lymph nodes. There were, for instance, clearly defined areas, nodules of tissue, which he has called germinal centres, and these were associated specifically with plasma cells. Furthermore, he was able to link this combination of germinal centre and plasma cell functionally with the production of antibody and gammaglobulin.

By means of steady development from this line of enquiry, comparatively slowly from the study of many cases of disease, from animal experiments, and from laboratory studies—very far in mood and fact from the dazzling moment of insight, the traditional "great discovery"—Robert Good has been principally responsible for building up the picture of the immune system working in two complementary halves.

Repeating briefly the material described in Chapter 3, this means that one-half of the system is controlled or influenced by the thymus, with small lymphocytes that emerge from the thymus being apparently responsible for the "information"-processing functions, such as recognising antigen and holding the "memory" of a previously met antigen. This half of the system is also responsible for what are called cell-mediated immune responses, such as the rejection of grafts, and some allergic and hypersensitivity responses. The second half of the system consists of the lymphocytes, which are primarily responsible for developing into plasma cells and for the production of large amounts of circulating antibody (and therefore also of gammaglobulins). This second half of the system is called "bursa-controlled" because in chickens an organ known as the bursa of Fabricius seems to play a similar controlling role to the thymus in the first half; the corresponding organ in mammals has not yet been defined.

Good believes that he was the first person to discover the key role played by the thymus in the immune system. This is a tricky point because there is fierce dispute among the immunologists as to who exactly can claim scientific priority in the discovery, the chief counter-claimant being the Australian Jacques Miller, who was working in London at the crucial period (1961–62). Discretion being so much the better part of valour I have no intention of trying to adjudicate on the matter, nor even of attempting to present the evidence on which adjudication might be made. The important point is that no one denies that Good and his colleagues in Minneapolis, Jankovic and Waksman in Boston and Miller in London, were all working independently and simultaneously on the same problem and came up with the same answer.

Up to the time of this discovery the role of the thymus had been a complete mystery—even more, it had been something of a puzzle, because the thymus, which is a comparatively large organ in the late embryonic and childhood stages of development, becomes smaller as the animal matures and appears to be virtually atrophied in old age. When it was established that the thymus plays a vital role in the development of the immune system, this change in size and even more its timing, was immediately seen to correlate with the discovery that immunological tolerance could be artificially achieved in the immediately prenatal and neonatal stages of development.

In principle, the role of the thymus was established by removing it surgically from mice in the neonatal period and showing that the treated animals could not reject grafts and had much reduced powers of making antibody. Experimental results before 1900 had in fact suggested that there was some difference between the "central" lymphoid tissues and the "peripheral" tissues such as spleen and lymph nodes. Many suggestions throughout the intervening years had followed that the thymus was an immunologic organ, but no clear experimental evidence for this had ever been found. We now realise that this was because the thymus is at the peak of its activity in the very first days of life and plays only a much-muted role when the animal is adult. However, Good had studied a male patient with a cancer of the thymus and noted that there were immunological symptoms. This, combined with studies by veterinary scientists on the removal of the bursa of Fabricius in chickens in the first days after hatching, turned people's attention to a possible immunological role for the thymus in the first stages after birth. Removal of the thymus at this time showed remarkable results: treated mice were rendered immunologically incompetent to such an extent that some would actually accept skin grafts from the rat, a totally different species.

But any tendency in the first excitement of 1962, to think that the thymus was *the* immunological organ was quickly checked. The situation was not so simple. The rabbit, for instance, did not show the same response as the mouse to what is clumsily called neonatal thymectomy—the removal of the thymus straight after birth. And of course the chicken, which had been shown by the veterinary people of Wisconsin in their significant experiments of 1954 and 1955 to suffer reduced power of making antibody when the bursa of Fabricius was removed, had a thymus like any of the mammals.

During the following three years it was clearly shown that the thymus, though of great importance to the immunological system, was not the sole controlling organ. Mice whose thymus had been removed immediately after birth would accept skin grafts from other individuals, and furthermore failed to produce the symptoms, like those of allergic reactions, which the immunologists call delayed hypersensitivity. They died young, they often suffered from a wasting disease and lack of growth, and there was almost always heavy infection. However, it was clearly shown that they could develop plasma cells and manufacture gammaglobulins and antibody. In this respect of antibody production they were not totally incompetent, just inefficient. And in some experiments it was shown that the secondary response to a particular antigen was even more depressed than the first response when the thymus had been removed. All this evidence points towards the thymus-dependent part of the immunological system being responsible for two main activities—the cell-mediated immune response, as in graft rejection and hypersensitivity, and the information, memory-carrying, and recognition part of the process.

For the sake of clarity it is better to add here, rather than in chronological sequence, that more recent experiments have shown that the thymus does continue to have some effect on the immunological system right through to late in life. Notably, it plays a major part in the repair of the immune system if it has been damaged by radiation, and we can nowadays demonstrate rather long-term, slowly developing weaknesses of the defences when the thymus has been removed in adult life.

But meanwhile, parallel and complementary work on the bursa of Fabricius (the lymphoid organ right at the end of the alimentary canal in chickens, only just inside the anus) was showing with increasing certitude that the bursa-dependent part of the immune system was responsible for the development of plasma cells and those tissues in the lymph nodes where antibody is produced. Indeed, it became evident that the actual populations of cells dependent on each organ could be separated and shown to differentiate at various times in the life history.

Nevertheless, there was considerable uncertainty about

the whole matter, as different theories were held by different groups of workers, and apparently mutually contradictory results reported. In particular, results for different species of laboratory animal seemed to show different mechanisms at work. This confusion now appears to have been caused largely because, under the influence of the thymus and the bursa, the peripheral lymphoid tissues of different species of animals develop at different times in the embryonic and neonatal life. From an experimental point of view, the way to solve this difficulty is to irradiate the animals as well as removing the thymus or bursa immediately after birth. This eliminates the peripheral lymphoid tissue and cells that have already developed under the influence of the two organs up to that time and enables clear results to emerge.

It is this clearing-up operation that has proved another major triumph for Robert Good's laboratories. The published results of the "irradiation plus operation" technique, outlined with his colleague Cooper, in a whole series of papers from 1965 onwards, have helped to clarify the situation. With another colleague, Peterson, Good's study of a particular disease of the chicken's gut lymphoid tissue showed quite clearly that this disease affected the bursa-dependent cells and not the thymus-dependent cells. By removing the bursa, the disease could be checked. Removal of the thymus made no difference; the two sets of cells, the two parts of the immune system, are dissociated. This is a typical Good strategy, using a comparatively rare disease as "one of Nature's experiments" and drawing conclusions from it about wider issues.

So there are two separate, cooperating halves of the immune system in birds, mammals, and man, one half dependent on the thymus; the other dependent, in chickens, on the bursa of Fabricius. The problem is that man and the other mammals have no bursa of Fabricius. So what organ in man plays the part of bursa to control the development of our antibody-manufacturing system? Or, to put it in a way that Robert Good might prefer, what organ has failed when a patient suffers from agammaglobulinaemia? The answer is that we don't know—an answer that is brutal, and, to me, rather surprising in view of the overall development of medical science. There are, however, several candidate organs. The appendix and the tonsils, both of which most doctors have regarded as expendable, have entered into the discussion, largely on the ground that the appendix of the rabbit has been shown to have an immunological function, though it is not yet clearly defined. There is also evidence that the intestinal tonsils of some laboratory animals may have some function in the development of the immune system. But the likeliest candidate organ, and the one which most immunologists would favor at the moment, is a rather mysterious set of pale patches on the skin of the lower gut. These are called Peyer's patches and their function is obscure, but they are almost certainly lymphoid tissue and have a broad similarity in location to the bursa of Fabricius in birds.

Another major problem still awaits solution in this field. The role the thymus plays in the immune system is now reasonably clear, yet it is still very far from clear what the thymus actually does or how it does it. Certainly, it seems that cells issuing from the thymus disperse to all parts of the body; some of these cells seem to come from the thymus itself, others seem to be cells coming into the thymus from other places (notably the bone marrow) and then emigrating to all parts of the body, presumably with their immunological competence improved or otherwise altered by their stay in the thymus. But we know that most of the thymus cells, small lymphocytes in very large numbers, never leave it at all. The job of elucidating the precise activity of the thymus has been tackled largely by taking away the thymus of mice at birth, and then trying to restore the missing functions either by grafting in lumps of thymus as a direct replacement or by injecting cells from other organs, such as spleen cells or lymph node cells.

One particularly interesting line of work was to take thymectomised mice and then put back into them thymic tissue. This tissue, however, was enclosed in very small chambers, made of material (Millipore) with pores so small that they would not allow whole cells to pass through, although chemical molecules could escape. Using this technique, mice whose thymus had been removed were able to recover from the wasting disease that invariably affected them and even gained some return of their ability to resist skin grafts. The work with these Millipore chambers implies that the thymus produces some hormone that makes the cells that leave it immunologically competent. There is supporting evidence that the bursa of Fabricius may also work at least partly by producing a hormonal substance, but neither thymus hormone nor bursa hormone has yet been identified or even isolated.

The broad outlines of the picture are reasonably clear, but a vast amount of work remains to be done to elucidate the mechanisms. However, the clarifying of the main picture has already allowed Good to define much more clearly the nature of human diseases in which the immunological system is affected. Within the last four years (1968) he has worked out the first classifications of the primary immunological disorders. There has been international confusion in this matter, similar disorders being called by different names in different countries. Thus there is Swiss agammaglobulinaemia, which differed from the agammaglobulinaemia that started Good on his immunological career, and which is in any case also called Bruton's disease. Swiss agammaglobulinaemia is also known as Glanzmann and Riniker's lymphocytophthisis.

There is Good's syndrome, Wiskott-Aldrich syndrome, and Mrs. Louis Bar's syndrome, Nezelof's syndrome, and Di George's syndrome. All are diseases of the immunological system. Most of the sufferers do not survive infancy; all are open to violent and repeated attacks by viruses, fungi, and other infective organisms; and in one way or another, all suffer from deficiencies in the defences that normally fight off infections and, even more, prevent second occurrences of the same infection. But in some of these diseases the number of circulating lymphocytes is apparently normal, in others there are virtually no lymphocytes at all. In some cases the thymus appears normal, in others it is missing altogether. In some cases there is apparently normal antibody response to antigens, in others there is no response to any antigen at all. In yet other cases of immunological disease there seems to be almost every possible variation between these extremes.

Based on the idea of two almost dissociated parts of the whole immune system Good has brought some order, some scheme of understanding, to the apparently hopeless confusion of the picture. By taking each reported syndrome and writing down the particular immunological deficiencies that characterise it, as well as those parts of the immune system which appear to be normal, the various syndromes can be grouped together. Thus there are those in which a failure of lymphocytes or plasma cells appears; those in which there are tissue failures, such as lack of development in the thymus or the peripheral lymphoid tissues; those in which there is failure to produce the normal amount of antibody; and those in which there is a clear genetic link, in that other members of the family have had the same disease. Then there appears a spectrum of cases—from the complete absence of a thymus at one end to an apparent complete absence of whatever may be the mammalian equivalent of a bursa of Fabricius at the other. Those in the centre appear to be failures in the interlinking of the two systems, or else it emerges that a particular syndrome is the inability to manufacture antibody, a failure right at the effector end of the immune mechanism.

This classification of a dozen different immunological deficiency diseases was put forward on an agreed, if provisional, basis following a World Health Organisation conference by Good, Seligman of the University of Paris, and Fudenberg of California in 1968. In the ensuing years a number of fresh categorisations of immune deficiency diseases have arisen. Probably about twenty are now widely recognised, though some of the different types are known by only one well-reported case; for they usually appear as massive infections and a child may well die without the true, underlying cause being revealed as a failure of defence rather than a successful attack.

Nevertheless, the importance of this classification of immunological deficiency diseases does not lie in a tidying up of medical nomenclatures or an international agreement; it lies in the hope of being able to treat the diseases, and this, after all, is the final justification of Good's philosophy of regarding disease as "an experiment of Nature." The cure of an immunological deficiency disease necessarily involves the reconstitution of the deficient system—the ineffective part of the system must be replaced in the sufferer. During the last couple of years the first such successful reconstitutions have been reported. A number of groups have managed reconstitutions, in particular, the group which transplanted a thymus, or at least thymic tissue, obtained from a "bank" of foetal tissue being kept by Dr. Humphrey Kay at the Royal Marsden Hospital in London, into a child born without a thymus in the United States.

It is hardly necessary to say that Robert Good's group was one of the first to be able to perform a successful immunological reconstitution. Their case was not that of a congen-

itally missing thymus, it was of something known as "sex-
linked lymphopenic immunological deficiency"—in other
words, congenital absence of lymphocytes. In these in-
stances, since the children have neither thymus-dependent
lymphocytes to recognise antigen and to reject grafts, nor
bursa-dependent lymphocytes to develop into plasma cells
and manufacture circulating antibody, there is a complete
susceptibility to infection from a very early stage in life.
Measles usually leads to fatal pneumonia. Vaccination against
smallpox leads to death by infection from the vaccinia virus
which normally induces protection. Compulsory vaccination
with B-C-G against tuberculosis, as practised in Sweden,
leads to death from infection by the B-C-G organism. The
twelve deaths recorded from 10 million B-C-G vaccinations
were all related to this immunological deficiency. This disease
only occurs in male children. For this reason it is described
as "sex-linked"; obviously it must involve some defect in the
chromosome which carries the sex-determining portion of the
genetic code. In families which carry the weakness genetically the chance of a male child having the disease is as high
as 50 percent.

In Good's first successful reconstitution case, the victim
was the four-month-old baby of a Connecticut family which
had already lost eleven young males in three generations
from apparently the same cause—a long series of infections
that the babies appeared to be unable to overcome. This
baby seemed to be following the same course. All the tests
carried out in New England pointed to lymphopenic immunological deficiency. It was actually a telephone call from
Meriden, Connecticut, to the University of Minnesota which
started the dramatic process; and it was decided to bring not
only the patient, but his parents and four sisters to Minneapolis. Once there, the diagnosis was confirmed and the main
problem faced. The problem was that the obvious way to

treat such a child would be to inject him with lymphocytes from someone else, or at least to inject him with stem cells from someone else in the hope that he would then be able to form his own lymphocytes. Earlier attempts to do this, including at least one attempt by Good's own team, had failed, however, because the injected cells had simply overpowered the defenceless patient with a massive "graft-versus-host" reaction. The most obvious way of repairing the immunological deficiency was rendered useless by the very weakness of the host.

But here the intensive research on organ and skin transplantation which had been carried out in other laboratories began to pay off. It had been discovered that there were certain antigens that particularly affected the success or rejection of transplants, the so-called histocompatibility antigens (more about them in later chapters). By matching the antigens found on white corpuscles (leukocytes) between donor and recipient, very much better success could be achieved in kidney transplantations, although complete identity between donor and host could still never be found. Even more to the particular point, studies by Simonsen in England, and by Billingham, now in Philadelphia, had shown that histocompatibility matching had a particularly strong effect in preventing "graft-versus-host" reactions. This was where the baby benefited by having four sisters, and why the girls had been brought to Minneapolis: the chance of finding a good histocompatibility matching with his own siblings was very much higher.

The baby arrived suffering from pneumonia, without lymphocytes, apparently unable to make any antibodies of his own, unable to reject grafts, and lacking tonsils, adenoids, and lymph nodes. One of his sisters did in fact give quite a good match for histocompatibility, but it was far from perfect. Her blood group was type O whereas the baby's was type A. But the case was desperate, so despite the worry about the non-matching blood the baby was given injections of white cells, separated out from his sister's blood, and of her bone marrow.

The first crisis came within a week: the baby began to vomit, became feverish, and developed a rash of a particular coarse type on his back and face. The symptoms were clear from the previous failures in reconstitution. It was the "graft-versus-host" reaction—the injected lymphocytes were attacking the baby's skin almost as though there had been a whole-body skin graft. Now this could be controlled by the sort of treatment normally used to make a graft acceptable. But the immuno-suppressive drugs which would have knocked out the attacking lymphocytes would also kill the bone marrow cells injected in the hope that they would set up a line of lymphocytes of the baby's own manufacture. On the other hand, if the work of Simonsen and Billingham had been correct, the "graft-versus-host" reaction should only be mild because the histocompatibility antigens of the baby and his sister matched, at least in the major details. The problem was that the laboratory work had been done on mice and there was no proof that man would react in the same way.

Good and his team recognised the moment of truth. In his own words, "We chose to gamble. We restrained our impulse to intervene and waited for the reaction to subside. It did." Within a week the "graft-versus-host" reaction, the fever, and the rash disappeared. At the same time, the first signs of successful immunological reconstitution became evident. Cells which could be shown to be female in origin, because they contained the sex chromosomes characteristic of a female, began to populate the little boy's bone marrow. The patient soon showed an ability to manufacture all the different types of immunoglobulin, and with them came, of course, the antibodies. Then a population of small lymphocytes began to appear, including some of the type which can carry out graft rejection and other cell-mediated immune responses—and soon the child showed that he could mount an allergic response, too. All the lymphocytes in the periphery of the child's body and 25 percent of his bone marrow cells were shown to be female in origin. In fact, it seemed that all the mechanisms for carrying out the immune responses were in satisfactory order. All that had been lacking was the lymphocytes. The factory sites had been in working order for making immunologically competent cells and proper antibodies; only the raw materials had been lacking. But the struggle was by no means over.

The next big problem came when the child showed all the signs of developing anaemia. All his A type blood cells, and the similarly typed cells that produced the blood, were being attacked by the O type cells of the donor. It was, in fact, another version of the "graft-versus-host" reaction: they had taken a child immunologically null but with normal blood-forming ability, and converted him into a child immunologically normal, but suffering from a severe damage to his blood-forming ability.

The only comfort was that if the patient had accepted a transplant of stem cells which would form immunologically competent cells, he might very well accept also a transplant of stem cells which would develop into blood-forming cells. So Good and his team gave their patient a second transplant of bone marrow cells from his sister. This time there was no "graft-versus-host" reaction. The first transplant had achieved a state of immunological tolerance. The child very rapidly started manufacturing red cells, white cells, platelets, and other typical blood constituents. The new cells were of female origin and of his sister's O type. Once again normal stem cells had been placed in empty "factory sites" and had duly developed and differentiated into exactly the type of products the factories were supposed to produce. Four months after the last treatment the child was virtually normal, with normal immune responses, and a full lymphoid system. But his bone marrow cells were female in origin and his blood was O group.

This example of reconstitution of the immunological system, and the parallel and virtually stimultaneous treatments of other forms of immune deficiency disease by other American teams, is possibly, according to Robert Good, the start of the era of "cellular engineering." We have heard quite a lot in recent years about "genetic engineering," and there are many people who are worried about the implications if ever this becomes a serious possibility. Cellular engineering—the replacement of whole populations of defective cells, or the introduction of lines of effective, working cells where previously there was nothing—seems to be a much simpler way of achieving the sort of results the molecular biologist dreams about in genetic engineering. It would also avoid many of the theoretical, ethical, and even political dangers which genetic engineering might introduce.

Cellular engineering is not, however, confined to treating immunological deficiency diseases. There is a clear perspective of ways in which it could be used to treat malignant diseases such as leukaemia, but that is matter for the next chapter. To sum up Robert Good's own philosophy about the connection between treatment and the learning of new things: "These patients have taught us a tremendous amount about how the body defends itself against infection, against foreign tissue. For us who have used these patients in this way it is a very exciting event to be able to return something to them by way of treatment." [2]

Chapter 8

The Importance of Immunology

The importance of immunology lies at present in three main areas—areas in which the problems and answers provided by the theoretical approach of the science of self can produce practical results and improvements of the greatest value, and where the demands for practical advances are likely to lead to increases in scientific understanding that are intellectually most exciting. The first of these areas is transplantation surgery. Here the powerful unconscious forces of immunity, unaware of the greater good of the whole organism, work to our disadvantage when we want to replace a damaged or useless organ with tissues from a not-self body. So we want to deceive or defeat our own immune strength—to make our own bodies "unself-conscious." The second important area is that of cancer. Here we suspect that our immune reactions are not good enough, that the surveillance system which normally detects not-self is being deceived when our own cells develop wrongly into malignant forms. The situation in this area is much less clearly developed but there is hope that we might work out a way of making the defences against not-self more discriminating and more active. Thirdly, there is the immunology of reproduction, centring upon what is at present the great mystery of why a mother does not reject the child which is so clearly not-self. Or, taking the question back further, why do females not reject male sperm, and is there a valuable contraceptive technique to be developed out of the answer to this question?

I propose to deal with each of these three areas in turn.

1. Transplantation

Most people learn of the importance of immunology through their awareness of the progress of transplantation surgery. Immunology has therefore become linked with transplantation in an incorrect way. The central problem of transplantation is an immunological problem, but the central problems of immunology are not those of transplantation. Immunology and transplantation are really two different lines of progress which have a common meeting point.

Heart transplantation, of course, has attracted the most public interest. Undoubtedly the emotional overtones of this particular operation, with the necessarily concomitant problems over the death of the donor, have given another regrettable twist of bias against a widespread understanding of the real problems involved. The medical profession, in Britain at least, strongly resents the publicity which has surrounded the whole story of the heart transplant. I will not deny that I have played a part in giving publicity to heart transplants, in "covering" the story as a journalist. I cannot and will not attempt to defend all the actions and stories of the mass media of communication in covering these operations; but I make no apology for the fact that wide publicity was given to them, and I believe the medical profession is unjustified in its demands for privacy or secrecy till after the event when it is bringing about such a revolution in clinical treatments. Revolutions of this sort, touching our deepest convictions and prejudices, involving problems of ethics which have never had to be considered previously, must be to some extent bounded and contained by broad public opinion and public approval; and this public acceptance can only be achieved by public information.

But despite the fact that public interest in transplantation only became considerable in the late 1960's, the history of transplantation stretches back more than one hundred years. The first transplant of a cornea, the transparent "window" in the center and front of the eye, was achieved in 1852, and such transplants have gone on ever since. The story of corneal transplants as a treatment for eyes damaged by injury or blurred by disease is well known and needs no retelling. All that need be said here is that corneal transplants have avoided the immunological problems of rejection because they *are* transparent, not directly supplied by major vessels of the circulation system of either blood or lymph, and therefore free from the visitations of wandering lymphocytes or antibody.

The publicity about transplants has concerned the transplantation of organs—large, solid masses of tissue like kidneys, hearts, and livers. In fact, the transference of any tissues, and cell-containing substances, from one body to another is a transplant. Taking bone marrow from one person and putting it into another, as we have seen in the case of the treatment of children suffering from immunological deficiency diseases, is a true transplant. So is a blood transfusion. Most people know that in a blood transfusion the donated blood must be of the same blood group as that of the recipient or death may result. Most of us know our own blood groups—we are "A" or "B" or "O"—and we possibly carry little cards stating what it is. What is not generally realised is that these blood groups are statements of the most active antigens carried by the red blood cells. If your blood group is O, your red cells carry a particular set of antigens. And if you are given a transfusion of blood in which the red cells carry a different system of antigens, your subsequent illness and perhaps death will be a rejection episode, an immunological response between your body and the not-self transfused blood, an episode of essentially the same sort as the reaction of a recipient to someone else's kidney. The task of discovering the main blood groups of human beings and the administration of matching blood in transfusions has been an immunological triumph. Yet the process is essentially the same, although it happens to many thousands of individuals, as the matching of a donor kidney to a recipient, which is now one of the chief activities in the process of ensuring a successful kidney transplantation operation.

Nevertheless, it is still true that the possibility of performing organ transplants as a clinical treatment became a serious proposition only after Medawar's experiments showing that immunological tolerance could be achieved. I have already suggested that organ transplants may have come about more quickly because of the coincidence that Medawar proved the point by using skin transplantation as his experimental technique. Sir Macfarlane Burnet has recorded that probably the first person to suggest taking any practical action as a result of Medawar's experiments was a young New Zealand surgeon, Michael Woodruff. He pointed out that if every baby in the first day or so of life were given an injection of its father's or mother's cells, it would later be possible to give the child organs from its parents if a desperate need emerged. Frankly, this was not a very practical proposition; its importance lies in the man who made it, now one of the world's leading transplant surgeons at Edinburgh University, the man under whose auspices antilymphocytic serum (or ALS, of which more later) was largely developed and under whose guidance one of the first lung transplants was made.

Within five years of Medawar's experiments, the first successful human kidney transplant was performed, based on surgical experiments carried out largely on dogs. In this operation the essential "immuno suppression"—the attempt to suppress the immune reaction of the body against the not-self tissues of the donated kidney, to prevent rejection—was carried out by subjecting the patient who was to receive the kidney to "sub-lethal doses of irradiation." This was based on results from early experiments and treatments with X-rays, and from the radiation sickness which had affected victims of wartime atomic experiments. It was known that X-rays, radioactivity, and similar phenomena, which we now recognise as a wide slice of the spectrum of all electro-magnetic radiation, (light and radio waves and infra-red radiation are other parts of the spectrum) would kill living cells, and affected circulating white cells, including the lymphocytes and other cells of the immune system, particularly severely. By subjecting the patient to irradiation by X-rays over the whole of the body but controlling the total dose of irradiation to a level below that known to be lethal, the immune system of the body could be put out of action, at least temporarily. Virtually all its "front-line troops" of active circulating lymphocytes and macrophages would be destroyed, while leaving the stem cells and germinal tissues almost totally unharmed. This irradiation treatment for immuno suppression did not in the long run prove acceptable or particularly effective; but it had at least enabled the modern technique of transplant surgery to get off the ground.

Why start with the kidney? The answer lies neither in the essentials of transplantation surgery nor in the essentials of immunology. There were two quite different reasons. First, the kidney is one of the few internal organs that come in pairs: it was therefore reasonable to consider taking one healthy kidney from a donor with two healthy kidneys to give to a patient who had lost the use of both his kidneys. In those days (although "those days" are only just over ten years ago) none of our modern techniques for taking kidneys from the bodies of people just dead and preserving them for the few vital hours until they could be transferred to a grateful recipient had been worked out. The second reason for starting modern transplantation with kidneys was "the artificial kidney"—the dialysis machine—had just been brought into operation. Its ability to perform mechanically the function normally performed by the kidney meant that failure of the natural organs no longer implied the immediate death of the patient, as failure of our single heart organ does. The machine won time for the surgeons, in which they could first consider and then apply the techniques of transplantation.

Successful immuno suppression was brought about, not by the sledge-hammer technique of total irradiation, but by following through one of the smaller points of the theory of immunological action that had been worked out in the research laboratories. A feature of the clonal selection theory is that a few of the small lymphocytes carry each possible version of antibody on their surfaces. When a particular small lymphocyte meets the antigen which matches its antibody, the lymphocyte is "triggered" into reaction; one type of reaction, the normal defensive type of reaction, is the immediate proliferation of the specific lymphocytes. In an earlier chapter I described how the proliferation of white cells on the chick-embryo membrane was Burnet's vital clue which indicated an immune reaction. Proliferation of the chosen defending cells is therefore an essential part of the immune reaction. The first really successful type of immuno suppression came from preventing precisely this process of proliferation.

The method of stopping proliferation derived from cancer research, in the shape of drugs discovered and developed with the aim of preventing the proliferation of malignant cells—cancer is essentially the uncontrolled proliferation of our body's mutant cells. This is but the first of a number of examples of the interaction of cancer and immunological research which will crop up in the following pages. At the moment the most commonly used of these drugs is azathioprine, a derivative of 6-mercaptopurine which was used for the same purpose of immuno suppression in the earlier days of transplantation. The exact mode of action of these drugs is not known, but it is presumed that they interfere with the manufacture of the nucleic acids, RNA and DNA, in the cells. The manufacture of these acids is a necessary preliminary to cell multiplication since the cell must double the amount of DNA it carries in order to provide a full set of chromosomes carrying all the genetic information for its daughter cell. Another commonly used immuno-suppressive drug is methotrexate, which similarly inhibits proliferation of cells by a different chemical method of blockage.

The use of corticosteroid drugs such as cortisone, which reduce inflammation, to treat rejection crises in the post-operative treatment of transplants is a normal part of the procedure when immuno-suppressive drugs are employed. Once the first thirty days are successfully survived, rejection crises become rarer and the patient is normally kept on a steady, or even slightly reducing course of azathioprine. This will prevent rejection occurring for two or even three or more years in the most successful cases. The converse of all this, as every reader of newspapers knows, is that the patient remains liable to infection by a wide variety of organisms that might otherwise be harmless, because his body's natural defences against infection are deliberately being kept in an inactive state. The continuous application of corticosteroids will produce other deleterious side-effects which are not so well known to the public, though the "moon-face" effect produced on Dr. Blaiberg in the last months of his life must have been seen by most people who look at newspaper pictures.

Clearly, the perfect answer to immuno suppression has not yet been found in drugs. The next major effort by the immunologists was the production of antilymphocytic serum, ALS. It was pioneered in Edinburgh (by members of Professor Woodruff's team, as mentioned above), in Boston, and at the Mill Hill laboratories of the National Institute of Medical Research in London. The idea was simple and completely immunological: if one injected lymphocytes from a man into an animal, for instance a horse, the horse would find them not-self and would mount an immune response against them, eventually producing large quantities of antibody against the lymphocytes, which would appear in its blood serum. Serum taken from the horse should then, if put into the man, attack the resident lymphocytes and thus reduce his body's power to mount an immune response against any invader, or against a graft or transplant. Casting back to the theory of how the immune responses work, the use of ALS will not, because it is specifically directed against lymphocytes, do much harm to the antibody-producing system where this has already been activated against invaders by previous experience. Nor will ALS harm the auxiliary systems of the immune mechanisms, such as the macrophages. The first experiments with ALS provided exceptionally hopeful results, because it seemed that the serum attacked principally those lymphocytes, the long-lived, thymus-dependent T-lymphocytes, which were most concerned with any potential rejection of a transplant. These are the lymphocytes carrying, admittedly, memory of previous invaders; but also the antibody to previously unmet varieties of not-self. They are therefore specifically the lymphocytes that will be trig-

gered by the antigen of a transplant. ALS appeared to leave
the bursa-dependent or antibody-producing, short-lived lymphocytes pretty much to themselves. It therefore seemed to
have good immuno-suppressive properties for transplants,
while leaving the normal defence mechanisms comparatively
unharmed. Thus it appeared to have a great advantage over
drug immuno suppression. It did not leave the patient open
to normal everyday bacterial infections.

ALS was used at first in small doses as an addition to drug
immuno suppression in human kidney transplant operations,
and, indeed, in some of the heart transplant cases. The results seemed excellent. But very recently grave doubts have
been cast upon its use. In some fairly large transplant centers
a closer look at the results achieved by ALS as compared
with those achieved with drugs alone have seemed to show
that ALS brings no advantage. Even more serious is the evidence that treatment with ALS increases the chances of the
patient developing cancer. Evidence from experimental animals treated with ALS shows a clear increase in cancers. A
glance back at the clonal selection theory explains why this
should be so. The lymphocyte system, the whole immunological system, is one of surveillance which is continually moni-
toring against the intrusion of not-self. A cancer cell, though
it derives from a self cell, has changed into a not-self cell. It
should be recognised as such and destroyed. There is, in fact,
according to Burnet's theories, reason to suspect that the immunological system may have been evolved as a surveillance
system against cancer cells as much as a guardian against
invasion from outside. Certainly, since cancer and immune
systems are confined to the vertebrates it would seem reasonable to suppose that both phenomena are connected in terms
of some evolutionary development. (Since the conference on
tumours in invertebrates described in the last chapter there
have been scientific reports of cancers or something very like
cancers—completely uncontrolled growths—in certain well-

studied creatures such as the Drosophila fruit flies; but these growths have been shown to be caused genetically by a fault in the chromosomes.)

ALS is now a highly controversial subject among those working both clinically and in research in the field of transplantation and immuno suppression. One well-known British transplant surgeon describes a recent conference in Glasgow as "the graveyard of ALS." Others, all over the world, are continuing to work on the subject. Throughout 1970 plenty of papers and reports appeared in the medical journals—one of the most recent came from Sir Peter Medawar and a colleague, reporting on experiments measuring the length of time of survival of skin grafts between monkeys treated with ALS. The report includes a suggestion that a degree of tolerance had been induced by treating the animals with ALS before carrying out the grafting techniques. Another line of approach which is the subject of current work is to use ALG, anti-lymphocytic globulin; here the blood serum of the horse or other animal which has been injected with foreign lymphocytes is further broken down so that only the globulin carrying the anti-lymphocyte antibody is used in the attempt to achieve immuno suppression after transplant operations. A team in New Zealand has reported encouraging results from the use of this technique. Nevertheless, it is broadly true to say that ALS at the present moment is somewhat out of favour.

At the moment the main hope of improving the results of transplant surgery lies in the techniques of "matching" donor and recipient. One of the most fascinating aspects of this development is that it is essentially an immunological approach to the problem, an approach based on the concept of the science of self, rather than on the more brutal one of trying to knock out a large proportion of the immunological defence system of the recipient body.

"Tissue matching," or "tissue typing," is based on the idea

that some people must be more "different" from each other
than others—antigenically speaking, "All creatures are
different but some are more different than others," to mis-
quote George Orwell. Within the virtually infinite variety
which the human genetic system allows among human beings, the structure of one individual's antigens, the molecular
flags on the surface of his cells which he himself recognises
as the symbols of self, must have varying degrees of similarity to the flags of all other individuals. In fact it is likely,
though not proven, that the nature of these flags or symbols
is a precise shape in three dimensions of certain molecules on
the surface of his cells. The shapes will be reinforced by the
precise positioning and strengths of the electrical charges at
the atomic level, and there will also be the normal chemical
affinities, valencies, and reactivities associated with the presence of atoms of different chemical elements. Just as two human beings, otherwise quite unrelated, are seen to be similar
in that they both have eyes of the same shade of blue, so can
two human beings be alike because some shape in their antigenic structure is held in common. Family likeness in facial
appearance is well known to all of us, and is the commonest
form of similarity we see. Antigenic likeness also occurs in
families for the same reason, that the common genetic inheritance of different individuals produces similarity at the cell
surface. But just as two sisters may look totally unlike each
other, so they may be extremely different antigenically. And
just as there may be a total stranger who looks remarkably
like you, so alike as to confuse and startle your friends when
glimpsed in corridor or restaurant, so there is probably a
stranger whose antigenic appearance is so like yours that his
tissues would confuse and even deceive your immune system
and its power of recognising not-self.

Historically, the line of research that established the existence of antigens on our internal tissues, now called histo-

compatibility antigens or transplantation antigens, sprang from cancer research in the late 1930's. And the apparently fortuitous connection between immunology and cancer is the sort of strand that now leads us to wonder whether the two subjects may not, in fact, be intimately related after all. The work was started by Peter Gorer in Britain and continued very largely by using the genetically pure strains of mice which were produced at Bar Harbor in Maine. There George Snell finally produced the clinching evidence of the existence of such antigens in the very early 1950's, though he continued to call them "factors" for some years after that.

Gorer's experiments used two strains of mice, one of which naturally developed a particular type of tumour while the other refused to be affected by this cancer. His method was to try to transplant or transfer the tumour from one mouse to another and his system was what we should now call the classical immunological research. We can interpret his results in the following way: The tumour-carrying strain of mice have an antigen which we symbolize by $+$, and a pure individual of this race, inheriting the antigen from both parents, is $+/+$; the opposite strain is negative for this antigen and a pure individual is therefore $-/-$. Mating between individuals of the two strains produces F_1, first-generation hybrids, which since they receive genetic material equally from each parent are $+/-$ for this antigen. Mice of this generation will accept grafts from either of their parents because they recognise the antigens of both parents as self. In the particular case of Gorer's experiments, all the F_1 generation could develop the particular tumour. Parents, however, cannot accept grafts from the children, because every F_1 creature possesses some antigen which neither of the parents possesses. In the next generation, F_2, obtained by mating members of the F_1 generation, classic Mendelian genetics says that a mating between $+/-$ and $+/-$ will produce offspring in these proportions—one $+/+$, two $+/-$, and one $-/-$. By grafting experiments between the grandparents and the second-generation offspring it is therefore possible to show that this relationship holds true. Gorer, using the tumor as grafting material, showed that it did hold true, and he suspected that in those cases where the tumour graft did not "take," it was due to antigenic or immunological incompatibility between the animals. He provided supporting evidence that antigens were responsible for the failure or success of the grafts in some degree, though it was nearly twenty years before Snell's work enabled us to give a firm interpretation to Gorer's results in the shape just outlined. The essence of Gorer's work was, however, to indicate that there were systems of antigens, determined by the genetic mechanism and operating at the cellular level in such a way as to make tissues either acceptable or unacceptable to the recipient body.

By now a great deal has been found out about histocompatibility (compatibility of the tissues) and the antigens that determine it in the mouse. No fewer than fifteen separate systems have been identified, and incompatibility in any one of these systems will cause a graft to be rejected. Even more complicated than that, it is guessed that each of these fifteen systems is determined by a different stretch of the nucleic acid in the mouse chromosomes—a different gene. At least twenty different varieties of gene—the technical term is allele—have been identified at just one of these sites, and one of these alleles is known to determine as many as ten specificities when it comes to expressing itself as antigen. There is a great difference in the effectiveness of these fifteen histocompatibility systems when it comes to rejecting grafts, however. Some are now dubbed "major" systems, others are "minor"; the major systems reject grafts much more quickly, as measured in days to achieve the effect, than minor systems. There are all sorts of interlocking relationships between the systems, in which they can mask or increase each other's effects. The full picture is very far from clear. But one thing *is* clear. There is one system which is much the most important. It is called the H-2 system, simply because it was the second histocompatibility system to be discovered. Complete incompatibility between two animals in the H-2 system will cause a graft to be rejected in as little as eight to twelve days. But here again two animals can be more or less incompatible with each other even at the H-2 system.

Now the importance of all this variation in compatibility, when it comes to transplantation operations, is that the greater the histocompatibility between two individuals, or the less the violence of the rejection, the less the amount of immuno suppression required to get a graft to survive on the recipient. It has been established that rats and chickens also seem to have one major histocompatibility system. It now appears likely that the same is true for man, too. In man the major system is called HL-A. In theory, therefore, it should be possible to carry out "matching" operations between potential donor tissues and potential recipients before performing human transplant operations. By securing the best possible "match," the graft should have a better chance of surviving with the lowest possible administration of immunosuppressive drugs. In fact, such "matching" is a regular occurrence nowadays.

Unfortunately, at least from the point of view of solving the problem of human histocompatibility in the abstract, it is not permissible or practical to breed genetically pure lines of human beings. Nor can patients or even volunteers be shipped round the world from one research laboratory to another to submit to lengthy series of experimental skin grafts. The process of establishing the outlines of the human histocompatibility system becomes therefore not complex but extremely detailed. The research (and for that matter the practical matching before transplant operations) is done with collections of white cells (leukocytes of all types) separated out from blood. Incidentally, the use of leukocytes, as the best carriers of tissue antigens, which seems eminently rational in view of our present theories of the working of the immune system, was discovered before the present theory was developed, as a result of one of Medawar's early experiments. Gorer's original work was done with red cells.

What has to be done is to find human beings who already possess antibody against the tissues of another human being. Serum is usually collected from women who have had more than one child and who have therefore developed antibody against their husbands' antigens which are present in their children. This serum is checked against samples of white cells from a large number of volunteers. Complement is added to enable the antibody in the serum to attack those cells which carry the antigens specific to the antibody. After giving time for the reaction to take place, a chemical dye called tryptan blue is added. The dye is taken up only by those white cells which have been killed by the antibody-and-complement. In practice, all this is done with very small quantities in little glass dishes looking like nothing so much as the rounded bottom portions of ordinary laboratory test tubes. But they are mounted in special racks carrying sixty or one hundred at a time. The experimental procedure leaves the scientist, then, with a hundred little pools of liquid varying in shades of blue, with perhaps some still quite clear.

But the subsequent operation has to be carried out again and again, with every variation and permutation of individual samples the laboratory worker can lay his hands on; and then, by a process of logical elimination exactly analogous to those demanded by crosswords and mathematical braintwister problems, a worker can sort out a series of different transplantation antigens among his samples and eventually prepare a set of sera which contain antibody specific to the particular antigen he has isolated. It must be admitted that the results and the testing serum are rarely quite so clear-cut and obvious as I have just made it sound. But they are clear enough to provide a satisfactory basis for practical tissue-matching work to support clinical transplantation operations in hospitals.

There are less than a dozen laboratories in the world which are considered to be in the top league in establishing human histocompatibility antigens. The group at Leiden University in Holland, led by Van Rood, was the first to make really great progress in the field and still remains at the very top along with the great American expert, Paul Terasaki. Ceppellini in Italy, Dausset and Batchelor at East Grinstead in England are other names in the top group.

The lack of really clear-cut definitions of particular antigens is shown by the fact that comparisons between the definitions of these different leading groups are not very precise. There are seven major specificities of the HL-A system which seem to be equivalent in the sera prepared by most of the leading groups. There are another half-dozen specificities where two or three of the groups agree with each other but which cannot be said to be widely accepted. Then comes a large selection, perhaps as many as fifty specificities, which have been found in individual laboratories but which have not yet been confirmed or agreed by comparison with other people's work. The confusion is in no way eased by the fact that each laboratory has formulated its own system of nomenclature for antigens and specificities discovered. Despite a number of international meetings no common system of naming or definition has yet been agreed. This is not at all satisfactory from the point of view of academic research or of forming a clear theory or pattern. All that can be said definitely is that it does seem clear that the general pattern of human histocompatibility is similar to the better-understood pattern revealed in the mouse.

Incidentally, there is a personal idiosyncrasy which seems to be shared by many of the immunologists working in this field. Most scientists, when they are trying to explain a point to a layman, seem to be driven to jotting down a sketch or formula on blackboard or scrap-paper. The commonest form of pictorial help is the graph; few scientists can resist the temptation to reach for a pencil and put down something like this: or this:

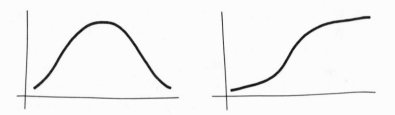

But immunologists have their own trademark. The drawing is often quite unnecessary for ramming home their point, but as with the graph it seems to help them to get out the words of the explanation. This is what the immunologist sketches:

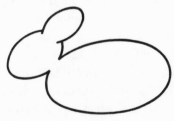

It doesn't matter whether you regard it as a long-eared mouse or a short-eared rabbit, they will inevitably put a skin graft onto it:

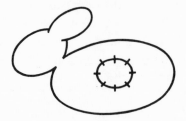

For practical purposes, however, the doodling characteristics of tissue-matching immunologists matter little, and the
differences between the various groups not much more. Any
efficient laboratory with a set of histocompatibility sera can
perform the necessary tissue-matching operations to a level
which is quite suitable for carrying out transplant operations. White cell suspensions are sent to the laboratory by
hospitals from patients who require a transplant, and the histocompatibility characteristics of a patient can be worked
out in terms of the sera available in the laboratory. When a
donor organ becomes available it can very rapidly be tested
for its histocompatibility pattern against the same sera and
the best-matched potential recipient easily discovered.

Because of the wide variety of human histocompatibility
and the comparative shortage of available donor organs, an
extra complication comes into the picture, however. Donor
organs may become available at one center—perhaps in Holland or Boston. It can easily happen that there is no well-
matched potential recipient there at the time; the best match
may well be a patient in Milan, Paris, London, or Philadelphia. Philadelphia is too far from Holland to allow a kidney
to be transported in the time during which it can be kept
viable outside the human body, although presently equipment is being designed with the object of keeping a kidney
viable during transport for as long as seventy-two hours. But
on a smaller, regional basis systems have now been established covering the Western European area and some groups

of American states. The histocompatibility patterns of potential recipients are fed into a central computer which then receives the patterns of donor organs as they become available and decides the best-matched potential recipient in its region. Jet transport gets the organ to the patient within the time limit.

The status of tissue matching and the hopes pinned onto its future development were well illustrated in the period of a single week in London in September 1970. The International Conference on Cardiology—the meeting of all types of heart specialists—was held then and one of the sessions was devoted to transplantation of the heart. Dr. Norman Shumway, head of the Stanford team of heart transplanters from Palo Alto, California; Dr. Botha, the immunologist and physician from Dr. Christiaan Barnard's Cape Town team; Professor DuBost, who has performed three of the French heart transplants; and Dr. James Mowbray, the immunologist from the British heart transplant team, all stressed their belief that improvements in tissue matching were being achieved and would eventually lead to better results. Within seven days one of the two leading British medical journals, *The Lancet*, published Professor Batchelor's results on a series of cases where skin grafts had been used in the treatment of serious burns. Good tissue matches, he claimed, not only prolonged the survival of the grafts but also contributed to the clinical progress of the patients. The other leading medical paper, however, the *British Medical Journal*, published a report by a South African team, from a Johannesburg hospital, which showed no correlation between tissue matching and the success of kidney transplants. In other words, out of a series of nearly thirty kidney transplants, there was no obvious difference in the survival time of the grafts between cases where the donor organ was well matched to the recipient and cases where the matching seemed positively poor.

It is worth noting here that, at the time of writing, there have been at least 170 heart transplants in the world, and the number of kidney transplants runs into the thousands. What is less well known is that there have already been more than 100 liver transplants. As a result, surgeons in many places, certainly in Britain, are beginning to face a shortage of donor organs. In many cases, doctors in centres which have not got transplantation programs are not sufficiently aware of the needs of their colleagues in the big kidney units when they have potential donor patients in the final stages of illness or accidental injury. Many surgeons in Britain hold that the press and the mass media are also responsible for the shortage of donor organs, because they have "frightened" the public by the publicity given to the marginal problems of transplantation and the ethical decisions involved (such as the decision about the moment of death of the donor). It has been difficult to get figures about the real seriousness of this situation until recently, and it is by no means impossible that the increasing number of transplants is revealing the true facts about a very small source of supply. But it has recently been stated that at Newcastle-upon-Tyne, where one of the larger British kidney-transplanting teams is based, in the first eight months of 1970 only six possible kidney-donor patients were notified to the kidney unit; in four of the six cases the relatives refused permission for the kidneys to be taken from the cadaver, and in the remaining two cases the kidneys were unsuitable, either because of disease or mismatching.

Another more personal problem looms up for the scientists. Some of the more distinguished of those immunologists who have pioneered the study of tissue matching came into the field regarding it as a research topic. More and more they have found themselves involved in the detailed and laborious work of carrying out tissue-matching operations for the benefit of their clinical colleagues who wish to perform transplant operations. Their research laboratories are being transformed into centres for routine analysis of histocompatibility antigens on a continuous, almost flowline, basis. Some feel they must get out and into new areas of research or else commit themselves to becoming medical production engineers. One of the new developments they are beginning to look at is "graft enhancement."

"Enhancement" just became known comparatively widely in the world of transplant teams and surgeons in exactly the week of September 1970 mentioned above, when an international conference on transplantation was held at The Hague in Holland. Enhancement was the subject that aroused most excitement, although historically it had been known as a promising development for more than a year before. Look, for instance, at the article on immunology by Dr. John Humphrey in the *Annual Report* of the Medical Research Council for March 1969 (I have referred to this admirable, clear piece of writing before). In the section on Transplantation of Organs, he writes:

> It has become clear from animal experiments that the recipient of a graft is liable to make an immunological response against any transplantation antigen represented in the grafted cells but not in its own cells. . . . Both a cell-mediated immune reaction (involving an increase in active lymphocytes) and an antibody reaction are evoked, but it is the cell-mediated immunity reaction that is generally responsible for destroying the grafted cells. In certain circumstances the antibodies may assist in this process but in others it appears that *they may actually help to protect the graft by coating the cells and preventing the access of the lymphocytes* [my italics].

Humphrey does not even use the word "enhancement" in an article intended to be read by laymen (or at least by those who are not immunologists). Only in the section entitled Future Trends does the word appear at all, when he says:

"Similarly 'enhancing' antibodies, which can protect against the effect of cell-mediated immunity and about whose nature insufficient is known, may be desirable under some circumstances but detrimental under others." This report, for a period running up to March 1969, was published in July 1969 and was therefore presumably written at about the beginning of that year. Yet by the end of 1969 the first reports of successful experiments using the technique of enhancement to give really prolonged survival of kidney grafts in large numbers of laboratory rats had appeared. In the first half of 1970 the technique of enhancement was being used in some clinical human cases, and, as I have said, in the autumn of 1970 excitement about the new technique really burst into the open at the Transplantation Conference at The Hague. This is a measure of the speed of movement in modern immunology.

To understand the workings and importance of enhancement, we must go back to the theory of how the immune system works. When a lymphocyte of the circulating, long-lived type meets the antigen for which its antibody is specific, it is triggered off into reaction and proliferation if the circumstances are right. We do not know the nature of this triggering-off process or the factors that decide whether or not it will happen. Nor do we know what determines the ensuing cell-mediated immune reaction or antibody-producing reaction or combination of both. What we do know is that there are these two different kinds of reaction, the cell-mediated type in which whole lymphocytes go into action and invade the tissue containing the foreign antigen, and the antibody-producing reaction described earlier. Possibly the chief distinction between these two reactions is the time scale. The cell-mediated immune response is rapid, violent, and comparatively short-lived. It also tends to be a "once-for-all" reaction, difficult to provoke again against the same brand of antigen. Large-scale humoral, circulating antibody production, however, begins more slowly, takes longer to develop, and lasts much longer. It can also be provoked again and again by the same antigen, and this is, of course, the normal basis for immunity. In terms of the reaction to an organ graft, it can be expressed like this:

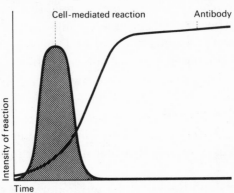

The cell-mediated immune reaction also occurs in cases of allergy and allergic diseases, and treatments similar to enhancement may be of value there too.

Broadly speaking, we do not know exactly how rejection happens; or perhaps it would be more accurate to say that many immunologists believe they know what happens at rejection, but unfortunately they do not agree among themselves. Some details of the mechanism are clear from microscopic sections of rejected tissues, and similar studies. It is clear that small lymphocytes invade the tissues of a rejected organ in large numbers. It is equally clear that there are also effects of the type we normally call "inflammation"—blood platelets, which are always rushed to the site of injury or inflammation carrying special chemicals and joining with fibrin to make blockages, can similarly be found blocking up the small blood vessels of the rejected organ. Still, the precise mechanism, the overall development, and the controlling factors of rejection remain obscure. In many ways this obscurity persists because we cannot yet observe a rejection reaction in process. Some things, however, are observable. Grafts which have not been rejected, observed when patients have died from some other cause, do not contain numbers of invading lymphocytes. Violent rejection episodes in patients who have received grafts appear to occur mostly in the first few weeks after the transplantation operation. In general, a kidney graft which has been kept for three months is likely to last at least a couple of years, and the longer it lasts the better its chances of lasting even longer as the rejection episodes appear to decrease in both violence and frequency. A similar critical point has already been noted in heart transplants at around the sixth month after operation. On the other hand, if the blood serum of a patient with a successful transplant is examined say a year after the grafting has taken place, it is found that his blood contains a high and steady level of antibody specifically against the graft. All this evidence goes to support the picture of the reaction against a graft shown above.

The object of the enhancement technique, then, is to mask or blot out the cell-mediated reaction against the graft by reproducing the conditions which we observe to obtain when a well-established graft has become a stable part of the recipient's system. Enhancement consists of doing what at first sight may seem to be exactly the wrong thing. Antibody is prepared *against* the graft and this antibody is given to the recipient at the same time as he receives the graft.

In practice it goes like this. Tissue is taken from the donor, ideally a large number of the donor's small lymphocytes, and is injected into some other animal. This "third party" mounts an immune reaction against the donor antigens on the tissue and produces antibody specific to them.

Serum, or even better just globulin, from the third party is then given to the recipient of the graft at and immediately after the transplantation operation. Further doses are given over the next few days. The recipient is thus "passively immunised" against the donor antigens in exactly the same way as was practised in the very early days of immunotherapy against infectious diseases. (Indeed, passive immunisation, the giving of already manufactured antibody, is still regular practise in certain emergency situations.)

The effect of enhancement treatment on grafts in animal experiments is certainly surprising—grafts have been maintained indefinitely even in animals given absolutely no immuno-suppressive drug treatment. The early results in a human case are reported to be very encouraging, too, though formal publication of results has not yet been reached. The interesting thing is that no one knows quite why it should happen.

The first hints of the possibility of enhancement came from experiments in transplanting tumours among laboratory animals in the late 1950's (cancer research again). It is assumed that the antibody delivered in the passive immunisation "homes" onto the donor tissues, arrives before the recipient body's lymphocytes, and by binding onto the tissue antigens of the donor organ, "hides" the foreign or not-self nature of these antigens from the patrolling lymphocytes of the recipient. Thus the triggering off of the recipient lymphocytes into the cell-mediated reaction mode is prevented. The only real evidence that this is what happens comes from the demonstration that the best results are obtained, in terms of graft survival, if the doses of passive immunisation are adjusted so that a small amount of the "manufactured" antibody is kept circulating in the recipient's system for the first week or two after the transplantation. The majority of the manufactured antibody certainly disappears from the recipient's circulation

shortly after it has been administered. But there is considerable mystery about the appearance of fresh antibody, manufactured by the recipient animal itself and specifically designed, again, against the donor antigens within a couple of
weeks of the transplant. The appearance of this antibody
does not seem to lead to the rejection of the graft, just as a
long-lasting graft seems eventually to be able to co-exist with
high levels of circulating antibody against it. Somehow the
enhancing technique manages to hide the not-self nature of
the graft until the danger of cell-mediated reaction is past
and the body has become normally immunised against the
donor antigens but tolerant of the grafted organ itself.

Snags may appear as enhancement is developed, but it
seems likely at the very least to be a valuable technique in
cases where complete immuno suppression is undesirable because of the danger of infection by other pathogenic organisms.

Finally, we come to tolerance. The long-term hope of the
transplantation enthusiasts centres on the possibility of artificially inducing complete tolerance in the recipient to the
tissues of the specific donor: that is to say, persuading one
individual to accept another individual, and no one else, as
being self. Medawar showed that such a thing was possible
under certain very particular circumstances. But these circumstances—the practicability of injecting the recipient
with the cells of the donor before birth or immediately afterwards—are plainly not susceptible of repetition under the
normal conditions of daily life and the clinical emergencies
of hospital and medical practice. Much of the most determined research by immunologists in the ensuing years has
been an attempt to find a way of making one adult animal
tolerant to the tissues of any other chosen adult animal.

The Medawar experiments can be interpreted in two
broadly different ways. Either there is some time at which

the immune system becomes mature, and any antigens introduced or presented to the system before that time will be
accepted as self; or the system develops over the whole range
of possible antigens, including self-antigens, and the enormous amount of self-antigen obviously present all the time
simply swamps those lymphocytes (and their potential descendants) which happen to carry the antibody specific to
the antigens of that particular individual. The second of
these alternatives is usually assumed to be the case because
it has been shown possible to achieve temporary tolerance in
adult animals—at least, a "paralysis" of the immune reaction
—by introducing enormous doses of some antigen.

The attempts to induce tolerance to a specific organ from
an individual donor in an adult animal have, therefore, taken
two different main approaches. The first is to attack the immune system of the recipient overwhelmingly the moment it
starts reacting to the foreign antigen. In practice, this means
giving extremely large doses of immuno-suppressive drugs
when the recipient receives the graft—and ALS is usually
added at the same time. This ought to affect precisely those
lymphocytes which carry graft-specific antibody at the moment they are triggered off into poliferation: the entire "family" of specific lymphocytes should be caught in action at the
first moment they identify themselves and their multiplication should be stopped. If this assault is effective, the treatment with immuno-suppressives can then be stopped and the
broader danger of lack of defence against other infections in
the months and years after the transplant will be avoided.
Although theoretically less satisfying, this method of approach to producing artificial tolerance has had immediate
practical effects, and is already influencing the methods of
treatment of day-to-day clinical cases of transplant operations in the hospitals.

The second approach is more subtle and difficult. It de-

pends on the discovery that certain common biological materials—especially the class of molecules called haptens—produce a particularly strong immune reaction. These can be
used in many ordinary immunological techniques as "adju-
vants"—added substances which increase the intensity of the
reactions. By taking suspensions of cells from the prospective
donor and extracting all the larger and more obvious structures by centrifuging, a fairly "weak" sample of the individual transplantation antigens can be obtained. They are mixed
with powerful adjuvant and the recipient is immunised with
this combination. In some way, as yet not clearly understood,
this deceives or distorts the reactions of those strains of lymphocytes which are specific against the donor and reduces, or
cuts out altogether, reaction against the graft when it is
afterwards introduced into the recipient. It seems likely that
there has been some competitive, selective pressure in favour
of similar lymphocytes against those which would be most
effective against the graft.

Unfortunately, much of this work seems unpredictable.
Techniques which have been successful with one particular
organ in one particular species of animal fail when tried with
different organs or different animals. The technique has certainly not yet reached the stage when it can be applied to
man, but the reports brought to the Transplantation Conference at The Hague in September 1970 have been described
as "encouraging," and *Nature* (September 26) admits that
"further studies along these lines may lead to predictable and
safe methods of making an individual accept an organ graft
without the necessity of prolonged treatment with poten-
tially dangerous agents."

2. Progress Against Cancer

The essence of cancer is that there appears in an individual a variation—a malignant strain—of his own cells that multiplies and grows uncontrollably until it disrupts the normal functioning of the whole system to such an extent that it is broken down and the individual dies. This is the common factor that enables us to classify a great variety of conditions under one heading; in fact, the outward appearance of the many different forms of cancer varies so much that it sometimes seems to cause more confusion than clarity to call them all by the same name. From the definition of the common feature it can be seen that cancer can occur at any point of any part of the body and can just as well be leukaemia—a variation in the circulating white cells (leukocytes) in the blood stream—as the growth of a large lump which kills by the apparently simple process of blocking up one of the main channels of the body. The malignancy of cancer lies in an uncontrollable growth of the aberrant cells. They multiply and proliferate far faster than normal cells, growing in directions that are undesirable, either penetrating into intact organs or pressing upon them. The surfaces of the cancer cells are more slippery than the surfaces of normal cells and the control which a normal cell exerts upon another normal cell simply through contact seems to be missing, too. But a large part of our problem in dealing with cancer is that we do not know how the body controls the rate of multiplication of its normal cells; we do not know how the body informs cells "which way" to grow; and we do not know how the presence of adjacent touching cells influences the behaviour of normal cells. It is obvious that there are many different ways in which different types of scientists hope to treat cancer. The pharmacologist and the biochemist hope to find chemicals which will poison cancer cells while leaving the normal cells unharmed; or to find some substance which is essential to the metabolism and multiplication of cancer cells and cancer cells alone, and then deprive them of it. The biophysicist and the biologist hope to find the parameters involved in surface contact between cells or in the directional growth of cells and then supply those factors that are missing in cancer cells.

Other scientists can search for the factors that caused the original variation in our cells and try to eliminate them from our lives. It is known that certain chemicals can cause cancer. It is more difficult to show either what precise variation they bring about in previously normal cells or how they do it. (It is lack of this sort of evidence that enables some people to continue to question whether smoking causes lung cancer; it is likewise lack of this sort of precise evidence that holds up campaigns to eradicate the causes of several industrial occupational cancers.) In animals some viruses cause cancers; that is to say, a particular type of virus injected into a particular species of animal will cause in many cases a particular type of cancer. It is assumed, though not yet proven, that the presence of the virus in a cell causes a change, a variation, in the genetic apparatus of that cell and its descendants. It can certainly be shown, not only that viruses cause cancer in whole animals, but also that viruses in cells in the test tube cause those cells to be transformed into malignant cells. No one yet has proved that a virus can cause cancer in man—largely because it is unacceptable to attempt to cause experimental tumours in men—though viruses have recently been isolated from human cancer cells.

The immunologist approaches cancer at a stage somewhere between those who consider the misbehaviour of the malignant cell and those who ask how the cell became malignant in the first place. He asks whether a cell that has become malignant has also become not-self. And if it has become not-self, how has it evaded the immune reactions which it ought to have caused?

It has not yet been conclusively proved that the initial variation in the cancer cell is a change in its genetic material, but there is considerable evidence that this is so. Certainly the presumption is strong enough to make it a viable working hypothesis. If the genetic change is enough to make the normal control mechanisms of the body ineffective, then that genetic change should be enough to be expressed exteriorly by a change in surface antigens of the tumour cell. There should in fact be "tumour specific antigens" (TSA) on the surface of the cancer cell. And so, indeed, there are. Once again the story of immunology is intimately involved with those genetically pure strains of mice at Bar Harbor in Maine, for it was there in the early 1950's that TSA was finally demonstrated to exist by George Snell, though the idea had been put forward more than twenty years before and then, for all practical purposes, had been discarded in the absence of techniques to demonstrate the validity of the idea.

Having demonstrated the existence of TSA, however, the immunologists have found no simple answers to the innumerable further questions that have subsequently leapt to mind. It cannot, for instance, be said that TSA are found on all cancer cells; nor can it be said that cancers of the same sort carry the same TSA, or anything this clear-cut. The proven existence of TSA, however, provides a firm starting point for planning further research aimed towards eventual clinical action. But before pursuing that line in more detail, let us look at some rather more theoretical aspects of the cancer/immunity relationship.

The extreme theory—Sir Macfarlane Burnet's—would relate the very existence of cancer to the existence of immune systems. I have mentioned this theory before; it is based on the fact that immune systems and cancer are peculiar to the vertebrate creatures, and that except for some rare cases of cancer, like growths in insects which seem to be caused by inherited genetic faults, neither cancer nor immunity can be found in invertebrates. It is therefore postulated that cancer and immunity may well have developed, at the least, simultaneously. Immune systems were developed against parasites and the very variability in cells necessary to achieve immunity allowed also the possibility of malignant variation. Subsequently, to ensure survival, the immune system had to develop to keep control of cancer and this survival value was, naturally, increased by the activity of the immune system against infections as well as parasites. Alternatively, the cell variability which is the root cause of cancer may have arisen as a side-effect of the greater differentiation in cells required by the more complex structures and functions of vertebrate bodies, and the immune system may have developed primarily as a defence against cancer. This may still be its greatest importance in our lives today.

Whatever one's attitude may be towards this theorising about the origins of cancer and immunity, the idea that the immune system is our primary line of defence against cancer is rapidly growing in strength, authority, and the number of people who hold it. This is often called "immunological surveillance," and it implies that we are all fairly continuously producing cancer cells. Each variation of our normal cells towards malignancy naturally occurs in one particular, individual cell for a start. From this one malignant cell a clone of daughter cells can develop, each equally malignant as it inherits the genetic change from the first. The job of the immune system is to spot such cells either as individuals or as very small clones; the surveillance system discovers that there are not-self antigens on the surface of these cells, antigens which reveal that there has been a genetic change away from the typical self pattern within the cell. The immune reaction is then mounted against such cells and they are normally destroyed. For a man or an animal to "get cancer" as a disease, with observable symptoms like a tumour, is therefore the result of a breakdown in the surveillance and destruction mechanism. A human patient with cancer has suffered a breakdown either in his surveillance system or in the immune reaction his body should have mounted against those cells which have mutated into malignant form. Those of us who do not suffer from cancer have been threatened with it many times, just as we have been threatened with infection from outside; but each time the threat has arisen, it has been spotted and destroyed by our immune system.

The comparison with a police force or counter-espionage system is unmistakable. The criminal, or traitor, has to be detected and rendered ineffective by the police force before his activities can become a menace to the whole community. This has to be done, however, without disrupting the activities of the main body of normal law-abiding citizens. But the criminal may escape detection by always appearing exactly like the law-abiding citizens. Or he may be suspected by the police and yet avoid capture and imprisonment by hiring extremely good, slippery lawyers and getting away with it every time (antigens too weak to provoke full immune response). A third possibility is that the police force itself is bad or weak.

I have called in this extended analogy because it will help to explain the various ways in which the immunologists hope to be able, one day, to improve the prospects of treatment of cancers. But by sandwiching the concept of "immunological surveillance" between a rather remote theory and an analogy I may have made it seem less down to earth than it really is—so here is some of the evidence for its reality

The evidence, once again, involves the use of genetically

pure, highly inbred strains of mice, where one individual is so like another that they might be identical twins; any one individual recognises the tissues of another individual of the same strain as self, and organs can be easily transplanted between one and another. If parts of tumours are transplanted, or injections of masses of tumour cells given, then an animal of the same strain as the tumour-bearing donor will accept them and the tumour will grow in the recipient. If the transplant is performed between different strains, then after a very short period of growth the tumour will be rejected. This shows that, broadly speaking, the tumour cells carry transplantation antigens that are the same as those of the animal in which they first grow. But by injecting animals of a different strain with inocula of normal tissues and cancerous tissues from animals of a donor strain, the recipient animals can be persuaded to make antibodies in the normal way against these inocula. If the antiserum from animals which received normal tissues is compared with that from animals which have received cancerous tissues, differences can be found. Indeed, antiserum from the animals receiving cancerous tissues can be reacted with normal tissue from donor animals until all the antibody against normal tissue is absorbed and there will still be antibody activity in the antiserum. This shows that there are extra antigens on the cancerous tissue.

Using cancers that have been caused by chemicals (carcinogens) and by viruses, it has been shown that it is possible to immunise animals against these cancers. Killed cells from the tumour are injected into a prospective recipient animal of the same strain as the donor. Any later attempt to transplant the tumour from donor to recipient will then fail, as the recipient mounts a normal immune response against the transplanted tumour cells. The experiment which really sparked off the modern interest in the immunology of cancer was done on these lines in 1951 by Prehn and Main, who used cancers caused by the application of the chemical methylcholanthrene. Since then it has been found that in cancers caused by viruses there are antigens on the surface of the malignant cells which are actually expressions of the fact that part of the virus genetic nucleic acid has been incorporated into the genetic material of the cell. All tumours induced by the same virus, whatever part of the body they affect, whatever the medical appearance of the tumour, bear the same antigen, the expression of the virus within.

(In some tumours of both rats and man, antigens have been found on the surface of the tumour cells which cannot be detected on normal adult cells but which can be found on tissues of embryos of the species. The finding supports the view that cancer cells may be cells which have "reverted" to the undifferentiated conditions of the earlier stages of growth.)

Very clear immunisation effects are easiest to demonstrate with the cancers caused by viruses or chemicals. Cancers which arise spontaneously, and which are normally slower growing, reveal much less antigenic activity. It is exactly what one would expect if the immunological surveillance theory is correct. It has also been clearly demonstrated that the immune system reacts to the transplantation of a cancer in exactly the same way as it reacts to the transplantation of a healthy organ. The cell-mediated reaction is what is important in rejecting a cancer. And, although circulating humoral antibody against the TSA is produced, this seems incapable of killing the cells of a solid tumour. Antibody can, however, attack cells of a non-solid cancer, such as leukaemia or marrow cancers, where the cancerous cells circulate individually. In fact, it can clearly be shown that the phenomenon of enhancement by antibody action can help to make a tumour transplant "successful": the recipient animal is first immunised with small doses or killed cells of the proposed tumour transplant, then the transplant of the solid tumour can be made when antibody is circulating in the recipient. This treatment will allow solid tumours to be transplanted from one strain of animals to another. Finally, it is easier to transplant tumour from one strain of animals to another by transplanting into very young recipients, just as this is the time of life, before the immune system becomes mature, when it is easiest to induce tolerance.

The corollary of all this is the depressing idea that the immuno-suppressive treatment, which is used clinically to help recipients avoid rejection of organ transplants, not only increases the liability of the recipient to infection by the pathogenic organisms which always threaten the human system, but also increases the likelihood of his developing cancer while his surveillance system is out of action. The possibility of ALS having a particular tendency to allow the growth of tumours—and therefore of its being on the whole undesirable for large-scale use in clinical transplantation techniques—was revealed by work on the general problems of TSA. The antilymphocytic serum was being used simply as a laboratory tool to help sort out the problems of the immunology of cancers, and its effects being compared with the results of cutting out the thymus in young animals. ALS is primarily designed to reduce the cell-mediated reaction by attacking lymphocytes. Injections of ALS shortly after birth were then found to increase both the rate of development of tumours and their rate of growth.

It is now being realised, furthermore, that even the normal chemical immuno-suppressives used after transplant operations are increasing the rate of cancer in patients. Some 4,000 people all over the world have now received kidney transplants. The latest figures show that some 30 of them have developed cancers, mostly of the lymphoid system. Whereas the prevalence of this particular type of cancer in the normal population is not quite 1 case in each 100,000 people, it has appeared in 12 out of 3,000 kidney graft recipients. This rate of cancer induction is far too small to be any indication against grafting operations, but it can be considered a significant pointer to the role of the immune system in preventing cancers under normal circumstances.

Now if it is true that most cancer cells are destroyed by the immune system before they have a chance to multiply greatly, and if it is correct that well-established, clinically obvious cancers exist only because their surface antigens are too weak to provoke a full immune reaction, then the immunologist ought to be able to devise some means of strengthening the immune reaction so that existing cancers will be attacked. Most people in the fields of both cancer treatment and immunology have come to accept that these deductions are true, and many immunologists are seeking ways in which they may be able to treat cancer sufferers.

A pioneer in this field is Dr. Avrion Mitchison, who worked with George Snell at Bar Harbor in the years when TSA were being definitely demonstrated. He now leads a team at the National Institute of Medical Research at Mill Hill in London, and we can regard his approach as fairly typical of the way many immunologists are thinking. The reasoning is that, since the TSA of an existing tumour is too weak to provoke the full immune reaction, it would be best to introduce new "strong" antigens onto the surface of the tumour cells. The new antigen, or determinant, is called the "helper." It is quite simple to stick some molecules onto the surface of cells by fairly well-known chemical reactions. If the molecules stuck onto the surface of cells are known to be of the right sort to act as antigens (and that means roughly that they are large enough biological molecules to provoke an immune reaction in their own right), the job ought to be possible. Haptens and several sorts of protein are not only known to be antigens, but can be stuck onto cell surfaces; and they are so well known in the laboratory, because they have been used for other investigations, that their effects can often be quantified. They are the helpers of choice. But it is also possible to produce helper determinants by other means, such as by introducing a known oncogenic (cancer-producing) virus into tumour cells. A population of tumour cells is therefore taken from a sufferer and the cell-surface determinant is put onto them. In the case of the best-known hapten, dinitrophenol, it involves little more than a straight chemical reaction in a test tube. The modified cells are then transplanted into an individual—a mouse of the same strain —who would normally tolerate the unmodified cancer cells. When trying to treat a human patient, the modified cells of his own tumour are transplanted back into him. The appearance of the helper determinants—new antigen—provokes an immune reaction in the recipient of the transplanted cells, even if the recipient is the original owner of these cells, now modified. But the reaction against the helper antigen also provokes increased reaction to the TSA which is near it on the surface of the modified cells. The lymphocyte lines which are specific against the TSA, and have thus been roused to greater activity, will then exert themselves against the TSA on the cells of the original tumour and destroy them.

There have been many experiments in the last couple of years putting these notions to the proof. Some have been research experiments performed with laboratory rats and mice, others clinical experiments performed with human cancer patients, notably in Detroit and Sweden. Some results have been encouraging, others much less so. The problem in interpreting the results and designing the next experiments is that no one quite knows what the helper antigens actually do. It is clear that in some cases the helpers really do help, in the sense that the original tumour is seriously attacked. It may be that the helpers somehow weaken the modified cells, and attenuate them in rather the way that bacteria or viruses are attenuated on purpose in attempts to make protective vaccines against infectious diseases. The immune reaction against these modified, attenuated cells might well also attack the tumour and be of benefit to the patient. Useful, but from the immunologists' point of view uninteresting. A variety of other mechanisms can be suggested. The helpers might provide a point of weakness on the modified cells; they might in some way take the modified cells to such areas as the lymph nodes, where the immune reaction would be strengthened by a localisation effect. Or they might, by their very presence on the cell surface, cause some change in the shape of the TSA on the modified cells, thus provoking a stronger reaction which is carried through to the TSA on the unmodified cells. All useful, again, but only of moderate interest to the theories of immunology.

The greatest interest will be aroused if it can be shown that the beneficial effects of helper determinants come about because they stimulate cell-mediated immunity reactions. This will also promise the greater chance of developing the technique to genuinely useful dimensions, because it is a cell-mediated reaction that we really want to provoke against a solid tumour.

There are a number of pieces of evidence which point to the fact that helper activity is part of the cell-mediated immune mechanism. It is known, for instance, that if a body is injected with a hapten attached to one protein, the body is immunised only against the "carrier" protein and is not found to be immunised if the hapten is then injected attached to some different protein. Yet if antibody against the carrier protein is prepared in some other animal and then given to a recipient, no helper effect will appear. Judged on the timing, too, it seems likely that the helper effect is part of

the cell-mediated immune reaction, for it appears very
shortly after immunisation and long before large amounts of
antibody can be manufactured by the recipient—and quick
reaction is a feature of cell-mediated response. Finally, in experiments where ALS has been used in conjunction with
helper techniques, it has been found that the results vary
very much according to the amount of ALS used and the timing of the doses. Since ALS, by attacking primarily the recirculating, thymus-derived lymphocytes, asserts its effects
mostly on the cell-mediated response, it would appear that
the differences in helper effect when ALS is also applied are
due to the helper activity being connected with cell-
mediated response.

What the immunologists hope to show here, although
they certainly do not yet have firm scientific evidence for it,
is that there is cooperation between the thymus-derived lymphocytes and the antibody-producing lymphocytes. They
suspect that the T-lymphocytes (the recirculating, long-
lived lymphocytes responsible both for carrying the immunological memory and for launching cell-mediated responses)
not only proliferate rapidly when faced by cell-surface antigens but actually pick up the antigen by one part of their
molecular structure and present it to the antibody-forming
lymphocytes in such a way as to stimulate the antibody lymphocytes (B-lymphocytes) into producing antibody and killing the antigen-bearing cell. The helper is believed to make
this process more active either by enabling the T-lympho-
cyte to "grip" the antigen more satisfactorily, or by stimulating the B-lymphocyte more effectively than the weak antigens of, say, TSA.

This at the moment is speculation. If it turns out to be
true, the study of the cancer/immunology relationship will
again have helped to solve one of the theoretical problems of
immunology, the problem of the relationship between the

two families of lymphocytes, the two arms of the immune system. And this new understanding would enable the immunologist to devise more effective ways, more effective helpers perhaps, with which to increase the natural immune reaction against tumours.

But it would not be fair to the immunologists to leave the impression that their efforts against cancer are all highly theoretical, aimed primarily at solving their own professional problems with the cure of patients as a mere secondary benefit. Immunological treatment of cancer has already begun. It has already scored some successes. One of the biggest programs of this sort has been carried out by Professor G. Mathé, of the Institut de Cancérologie et d'Immunogénétique, at the Villejuif Hospital just outside Paris. Reporting as recently as the end of 1969 in the *British Medical Journal*, Professor Mathé, already famed as one of the world's leading experts on radiation, radiation injuries, and the bone marrow, tackled twenty patients suffering from a particular variety of leukaemia (cancer of the white cells). He reasoned that the immunological approach would work best when the number of cancerous cells had been reduced as far as possible. So all the patients were given complete treatments with those chemicals which are known normally to kill white cells, the use of these chemicals to keep the number of leukaemic cells down being at present virtually the only way of dealing with leukaemia, which is usually a rapidly fatal disease. When as many of the leukaemic cells as possible had been killed, Professor Mathé started the immunological treatment.

To some of his patients he gave continuous administrations of B-C-G—the attenuated variety of the organism that causes tuberculosis, the substance nowadays regularly used for vaccinations against tuberculosis (see Chapter 2). Every fourth or eighth day they received a fresh dose, the ob-

ject being simply to stimulate the immune system generally, or non-specifically. To other patients he gave injections
of large numbers of killed leukaemic cells collected from a
pool of sufferers from the disease. Yet another group of patients was given both the B-C-G treatment and injections of
leukaemic cells. Finally, there was a group of control patients
given nothing except the standard drug treatment of chemotherapy. To understand his results it must be explained that
the standard drug treatment usually works for a while with
all patients, but as the unkilled, surviving cancerous leukaemic cells multiply at their uncontrolled rate, the patients
eventually usually "relapse." It is virtually impossible to
prove that a leukaemia patient is finally "cured" in the normal sense of being completely free of the disease; the effect
of treatment can only be measured by the length of time before a "relapse" occurs.

In Mathé's study all the patients on the standard chemical therapy relapsed at about the usual time. Just over half
the patients given immunotherapy also relapsed, most of
them quite soon in the treatment, shortly after their chemotherapy course was finished. (Possibly this is another indication of the cell-mediated response failing.) Four patients appeared to do well for a longish while and then had relapses at
various points ranging from seven months to two and a half
years after the end of the chemical treatment. But one patient is still alive and well after more than three years of the
immune treatment; four have survived without relapse for
more than two years. The total of those who have managed
to avoid a relapse for over a year and are still on the immunotherapy treatment is as high as seven out of the twenty on
whom it has been tried.

Perhaps the most important point about Mathé's treatment is that it illustrates the general method by which immunology is most likely to be brought broadly to bear on the

cancer problem. Until the major theoretical problems of immune surveillance and its workings are solved, it is widely felt that the clinical advances are likely to lie in the treating of tumours by standard modern practice—that is, surgery, radiation, chemotherapy—to kill the majority of the tumour cells and then bring in immunotherapy to finish off the job. The problem with modern treatments for tumours—the same problem as in leukaemia—is that it is virtually impossible to be certain that all the tumour cells have been removed or killed by drugs or radiation. And as long as any of the cancerous cells are left in the body, they may well start multiplying again. But a few scattered cells are precisely what the immune system ought best to be able to cope with, because that is its natural role in immuno surveillance. So this is most likely to be the way in which immunologically based treatments will come into large-scale use in the treatment of cancer.

3. Immunology and Reproduction

A baby initially appears flatly to contradict the theory of the science of self. It is a successful transplant performed without the aid of surgeon or immunologist. It is certainly foreign, not-self, to its mother: half of its genetic nucleic acid comes from the father and is expressed on the surface of the baby's cells as antigen foreign to the mother. Animal experiments have shown that a normal newborn baby will reject skin grafts from its mother and the mother will reject skin grafts from the newborn baby. So why did not the mother reject the baby in the womb?

Indeed, we can go farther back in the process and ask why does not the mother reject the father's sperm? The normal sexual process involves the introduction into the female body of a large amount of totally foreign material; both sperm and the prostatic fluid in which it is ejaculated from the male ought to be quite capable of arousing an immune response from the body of any healthy woman. Yet apparently this does not occur. Why not?

There are no answers to these questions at present. Or rather, there are a number of possibilities, none of which has much firm scientific foundation. But the task of finding out which possible answer is correct is not only exciting for both immunologists and physiologists, but may also prove of great value when applied to areas of practical interest. In the solution of these problems of immunology and reproduction and their practical applications the third great importance of modern immunology is found.

Obviously, the transplant that is a baby is privileged in some way to remain largely immune from the operations of the immune system. Presumably there is some sort of barrier built up between the mother and the foetus, across which the mother's immune system cannot operate. But when this presumed barrier is examined more closely its operation is seen to be highly selective, and the nature of its construction becomes highly speculative. Because this barrier *does* let immunoglobulins—that is, antibodies—cross from the mother to the child. This is certainly true of the most common type of antibody, IgG, the normal antibody against infectious disease organisms; most people know that a baby carries some immunity against infectious diseases for the first nine months or year of its life. If the mother has had measles herself, she normally passes on her measles antibody to her child and the baby has some protection in the early phase. Broadly speaking, it seems as if this mechanism is an evolutionary development to "cover" the period until the child's own immune system is mature enough to cope with invaders. But in certain cases, examined in more detail later, maternal antibodies cross the barrier and actually attack the infant's cells.

Furthermore, cells from the foetus can cross the barrier

and enter the mother's blood stream—this is especially true of red and white blood cells and it occurs most commonly during labour. But it can occur before, especially during episodes of bleeding which tend to arise in those women who suffer from high blood pressure, particularly during the last six weeks of pregnancy. The barrier seems, then, to be principally involved in preventing transplantation antigens from crossing from the baby to the mother, and lymphocytes from passing from the mother to the child, in such a way that a cell-mediated immune reaction against the baby can be prevented. But the actual evidence for this statement is non-existent, shaky, or even contradictory. Recent research, however, appears to show that there is some sort of barrier physically existing on the mother's side of the foetal tissue—possibly a layer of the large molecules called muco-polysaccharides, which are fairly common in biological structures.

I have called a baby a successful transplant, and we know that a transplant in some respects resembles a cancer—at least from the point of view of the immune system. Some very exciting work has started recently which is essentially following up this angle. The small group of cells that has developed from a fertilised ovum in a mammal's womb eventually implants itself into the wall of the womb. There it behaves at first very much like an invasive cancer. Furthermore, at this stage it avoids provoking the immune reaction of the mother, and this is the stage at which immunological surveillance might be expected to operate. If that small group of cells that represents the very first stages of an embryo is taken out of the womb of the mother, its natural home, and is transplanted to some other site in the body of its host, or even into the body of another animal altogether, it will behave at first just as it does in the womb—that is to say, like an invasive cancer tissue. It is, for instance, possible to grow the early stages of a mouse embryo in the testicle of a male mouse, or in the kidney cells of its true mother. In all these cases the group of rapidly multiplying cells seems to preserve itself against the immune reaction of the host tissue. It is possible that this is achieved by the growing embryo surrounding itself with a layer of specially protective, transparent tissue. The question immediately springs to mind: Is this how a growing cancer manages to survive? The elucidation of the details of this process is obviously significant for immunology, cancer research, and physiology and embryology. Among the pioneers of this work were the famous French scientist André Lwoff and a brilliant young Englishman at Oxford, David Kirby, who died tragically after a car accident, only a couple of years ago.

But some practical achievements have also been made. We do not yet know why a woman does not reject male sperm, but a very small proportion of infertile women who seek medical help have, in fact, been found to react immunologically against their husbands' sperm, and they have been helped by immuno suppression to conceive the children they want. This may seem a very small success, as so few patients have been helped. Its significance is instead that it opens up the possibility of achieving immunological contraception. There seems no reason in theory why a woman should not be artificially sensitised or immunised against her own husband or, just possibly, against men in general. A few scientists are already working on this problem. The advantages over the various forms of chemical contraception which are now much in vogue are likely to lie in the lack of danger from side-effects and the long-lasting contraceptive action of a single short treatment. The problem might be whether the effect was reversible; in other words, could the woman be made receptive to her husband's sperm again if she wished, or when she wanted her next child? But this is probably far in the future.

Nearer at hand and for the moment much more practically useful is a technique developed by the immunologists which has its greatest application in the clinical diagnosis and treatment of reproduction problems.

By establishing the concept of antibody, with its extraordinary specificity for one particular type of molecule, the immunologist has provided other biological scientists with an exceptionally fine tool. They can now identify extremely small amounts of biological material even when it is mixed up in complexes of the large kinds of molecules such as typify the living creature. The techniques of "radioimmuno-assay" in particular have been of great value to the physiologist in identifying and sorting out the hormones.

Hormones are the chemical messengers of the body. They are produced at many points—at the base of the brain, by the various endocrine organs, by the reproductive organs—and they circulate via the blood stream to the various target organs which they stimulate into the appropriate activity with a high degree of specificity. Extremely small quantities of hormone can produce major changes in bodily activity. In women the presence of a hormone, chorionic gonadotrophin, in urine is a sign of pregnancy. Once this hormone had been isolated, a quick and easy pregnancy test became available. Some of the hormone is used for injection into rabbits to produce an antiserum. Further hormone is coated onto killed and stabilised red blood cells. Mixing the anti-hormone antiserum with the hormone-treated blood cells produces an agglutination effect: the antibodies clump the blood cells when they bind to the hormone on the surface of the cells. But if "free" hormone, such as can be found in the urine of pregnant women, is added to the mixture, then the antibodies will bind to this free hormone in preference to the cell-bound hormone, and the cells will not be agglutinated. Furthermore, this action is quantitative; the amount of "haemagglutination-inhibition" is directly proportional to the amount of free hormone present in the urine sample. This technique can detect as little as 20 to 40 units of hormone in a litre of urine, where the earlier, purely biological Friedmann test needs between 1,000 and 2,000 units of hormone per litre of urine to give a definite positive result for pregnancy.

Radioimmuno-assay can prove forty times more sensitive even than the immunological pregnancy test. Indeed, it is now the method of choice for determining many hormones, for example, growth hormone or gastrin in clinical situations. Of course, the endocrinologists and doctors have to isolate some quantities of the hormone first. This material, or perhaps samples of the same hormone recovered from animals, is used to prepare antiserum, probably in guinea-pigs, which produce very good antibodies against hormones. Further hormone is "labelled" by the insertion into it, or addition to it, of radioactive atoms. A known quantity of the labelled hormone and a known quantity of the antiserum is then added to the human serum which is to be tested for the presence and quantity of the hormone. The antiserum will bind to labelled and unlabelled hormone in the test specimen in the proportion in which the two varieties of hormone are present. The combination of antibody and hormone will precipitate and this precipitate can then be isolated from the mixture. By measuring the radioactivity, the amount of labelled hormone in the precipitate and the amount of unlabelled hormone present in the original sample can be calculated with extreme accuracy. As little as 3 micromicrograms of a hormone can be identified by radioimmuno-assay, which has now also become a popular way of measuring the amount of insulin present in the blood stream in cases of diabetes.

In general, antibodies can be used by research workers to track down the presence of any number of enzymes, hormones, and other biological substances. By using antibodies labelled with fluorescent dye, the hormones and enzymes can even be traced to the organs in which they are being produced or in which they are working.

But the greatest achievement of immunology in the field of reproduction has been the discovery of how to overcome "haemolytic disease" of the newborn. The term "haemolytic" is used because the chief feature of the disease is the "lysis" or breaking up and killing of the baby's blood cells. But the disease is better known to most of us as "Rhesus baby" or, as it was once called, "jaundice of the newborn."

The problem arises when a woman with Rhesus-negative blood is married to a husband with Rhesus-positive blood. Rhesus-positive and -negative simply describe the presence or absence of certain antigens which are found on blood cells, very similar to the familiar ABO blood groups. The vast majority of people have the Rhesus antigen and the number of Rhesus-negative women is quite small: in Britain, for example, 64,000 women are estimated to run the risk of the "Rhesus baby problem" in each year out of a population which produces roughly 800,000 births a year. However, if in any pregnancy a Rhesus-negative woman carrying a baby which has Rhesus-positive blood inherited from its father should get any of the baby's blood cells into her blood stream, she will become immunised against the Rhesus factor and will produce antibody against it. In a subsequent pregnancy the anti-Rhesus antibody which is now in the mother's system can cross the "barrier" in the placenta and start attacking the blood cells of the baby while it is still in the womb. The attack on the baby's blood cells can be more or less serious. It can threaten the baby with death before it is born or it can result in only slight jaundice. It is quite common for the baby to need to have all its own blood drawn off and to receive massive transfusions of fresh blood immediately after birth. This fresh blood will keep the baby going until the antibody from the mother ceases to be active; then the baby can rebuild its own blood supply.

Of course this does not happen in every case of a Rhesus-positive baby born to a Rhesus-negative mother. Indeed, it can only happen in second and subsequent pregnancies, because blood from the baby of a previous pregnancy is needed to immunise the mother. In any case, blood cells from a baby do not always enter the mother's blood stream; this only occurs during bleeding episodes or during labor when the placenta is torn or ruptured. The chance of the mother becoming immunised at all is only 1 in 10. And there is a further protection in about 20 percent of the cases where a Rhesus-negative mother is in danger of being immunised against the Rhesus-positive blood of her baby. These are the cases where the mother's blood is even more incompatible with her baby than just a Rhesus incompatibility. If the mother's blood is incompatible with the baby's at the much stronger ABO blood groups, then the baby's blood cells which enter the mother's blood stream are destroyed before the Rhesus immunisation can occur.

It was these comparatively rare cases of natural protection against what is technically termed "iso-immunisation" that provided the clue to a way round the problem. The terms "Rhesus-positive" and "Rhesus-negative" are rather an oversimplification. There are several slightly different ways in which our blood can fall into either of these categories. The basic cause of this is that the Rhesus factor is not controlled by a single gene in our make-up but rather by several linked genes. And the action of these genes is linked with the action of the sex-determining genes, in addition to the possibility of there being "cross-overs" of the genetic material among the linked genes when a new individual is formed (i.e., when the nucleic material of a sperm and an ovum combines).

A group of medical researchers in Liverpool, led by Professor C. A. Clarke, was studying the genetics of butterflies for reasons totally unconnected with Rhesus babies. Among the females of the species *Papilio memnon* there are two common types: one has no tail, a black body, and a large white blob on the hind wing; the other has a tail, a yellowish body, and a small white blob on the hind wing. Experiments had shown that the second type was genetically dominant and it seemed that a single gene could convert the first type into the dominant second form. But every so often there appeared a third type of female, which had a tail, a black body, and a small white blob. There were in fact linked genes and not a single gene involved in the production of the final characteristics. Furthermore, the linked genes interacted with the sex genes because males of this species are totally different to look at. The hint to Professor Clarke was a hint by analogy; if the butterflies inherited appearance in the same way that human beings inherited Rhesus factor, we should be able to combat iso-immunisation also by mimicking nature. Incompatibility in ABO blood groupings destroys the Rhesus-positive cells from the baby before they have time to immunise the mother. He would mimic incompatibility. So now a Rhesus-negative mother who gives birth to a Rhesus-positive child is immediately injected with anti-Rhesus antibody prepared in someone else's body. This antibody kills the baby's Rhesus-positive blood cells before they have time to immunise the mother, and at her next pregnancy the mother has no anti-Rhesus antibody of her own to destroy her child's blood. The injection of anti-Rhesus antibody cannot hurt the first child because it has already been born before the mother is given the injection; nor can it hurt the mother because she is Rhesus-negative.

Naturally there was a great deal of work between the coming of the idea and the ability to put it into general clinical use. First Professor Clarke found some male volunteers and tried out the whole technique on them. The men were Rhesus-negative; they were given Rhesus-positive blood and then immediately anti-Rhesus antibody. In most of the cases it worked: the men were not immunised against the Rhesus factor on the Rhesus-positive blood. Then came the first clinical trials. Alternative cases of Rhesus-negative women having Rhesus-positive babies for the first time were given anti-Rhesus antibody immediately after the birth. The injected antibody should be eliminated in a few months, so the test of success was to see whether the mothers had anti-Rhesus antibody in their blood stream after the end of the artificial antibody should have come about—that is, were they or were they not producing their own anti-Rhesus antibody which could harm a later baby? The best that was hoped for was that 75 percent of the women would be protected by the new technique. In fact, the first results showed nearly 100 percent protection.

There was still the possibility that the giving of the "passive" antibody might simply have masked the fact that the mothers had nevertheless become immunised by the Rhesus factor; the only final proof would come when they had subsequent pregnancies. But all has gone well. Up to now the treatment has almost always proved successful and has been taken up by many other medical centers. Incidentally, a directly parallel and quite independent line of research was followed from an almost simultaneous discovery of the same principle in the United States in 1967, where the first groups into this field were at Columbia and Cornell in New York and at Long Beach in California. The American results, and figures from Germany, all confirm the promise of the treatment.

One big practical problem remains. Since it is extremely difficult to tell whether a Rhesus-negative mother has or has not received any blood cells from her Rhesus-positive child, the ideal would be to give them all this injection immediately after the birth of their babies. But to pursue this would mean producing a very large quantity of anti-Rhesus antibody, and the only suitable place for doing so is in the bodies of Rhesus-negative males. This involves injecting male volunteers with Rhesus-positive blood and then taking serum from them. There is a slight but calculable risk to the volunteers that they might contract serum hepatitis (infective jaundice) in the process. This raises ethical problems and various official working parties are looking into the practical problems.

But the problem of Rhesus babies should not be with us much longer. Immunology can chalk up one important practical advance in the field of reproduction, even if the immunologist must admit that his science has generally uncovered more problems than solutions when it faces that apparently privileged creature, the human baby.[1]

Chapter 9

The Disadvantages of Immunity

To the historian, "a Whig interpretation of history" means the cardinal fault of looking at history from the point of view of the present. It interprets the past as a series of struggles between progressive, right-minded movements, which can clearly be seen to favour the development of the finer features of our contemporary civilisation, and reactionary forces, which, however noble the individuals who supported them and however justified their claims at the time, can now be seen to be retrograde in purpose simply because they have not produced our present systems and mores. I would have to plead guilty to presenting "a Whig interpretation of evolution," at least as far as the immune system and the science of self is concerned. The development of defensive immune mechanisms against microbial invasion or against the internal disruption of cancer has been treated as something advantageous because we now feel it to be advantageous. But this is a self-centred point of view.

It is more realistic to view ourselves as being what we are because the immune system happened to develop in the way it did. A change occurred in one of the long spiral molecules which we now regard as being our inheritance. This resulted in that particular spiral molecule being able to hold on to the chemical material it had gathered about it and to prevent other spiral molecules from taking it away. In turn, the changed spiral molecule gained an advantage over very similar unchanged spiral molecules, which can be interpreted by saying that mammals or vertebrates with this particular immune system survived longer to breed more than those without it. We only know that that particular change was advantageous because it survived. In fact, the word "advantageous" means advantageous for survival. We are not the winners in some long race, we are simply the survivors. The immune system that enables us to survive better than some possible alternatives has not been designed in order that we may live. It has simply happened and its overall advantage outweighs its overall disadvantage. So far, we have looked at its advantageous aspects. Let us now look at the other side of the coin and see that it only appears to be another side: that it is the same mechanism and that its features, which we call allergy, hypersensitivity, and delayed-type hypersensitivity, simply shade across a spectrum into what we now see as "advantageous."

Allergy

Presumably human beings have always experienced and known about asthma, hay fever, the itchy rashes which medicine calls urticaria, and the strange way in which some individuals come out in rashes or suffer even worse disabilities after eating shellfish. But the first indication that all these things were connected and were basically immunological phenomena came right at the start of the present century. In 1902 two French scientists, Portier and Richet, were guests on the luxury yacht of Prince Albert of Monaco cruising in the Mediterranean—these were the high, golden days of Edwardian splendour when Monte Carlo was at the height of its fame. Possibly because his sea-bathing activities had been disturbed by the creatures, Prince Albert suggested that Portier and Richet should study the production of poison by the jelly fish known as Portuguese Man-o'-War, technically *Physalia*. There and then, aboard the Prince's yacht, the two scientists began their experiments and were very soon able to show that an extract from the long wavy filaments of the jelly fish was extremely toxic to ducks and rabbits. But when they got back to France they could no longer obtain specimens of *Physalia*, and Richet, in particular, turned his attention to the study of the tentacles of the sea-anemone, *Actinaria*. In Richet's own words this is how the discovery of hypersensitivity came about:

> While endeavouring to determine the toxic dose of extracts, we soon discovered that some days must elapse before fixing it; for several dogs did not die until the fourth or fifth day after administration or even later. We kept those that had been given insufficient to kill in order to carry out a second investigation upon these when they had recovered. At this point an unforeseen event occurred. The dogs which had recovered were intensely sensitive and died a few minutes after the administration of small doses. The most typical experiment, that in which the result was indisputable, was carried out on a particularly healthy dog. It was given at first 0.1 ml. of the glycerine extract without becoming ill: twenty-two days later, as it was in perfect health, I gave it a second injection of the same amount. In a few seconds it was extremely ill; breathing became distressful and panting; it could scarcely drag itself along, lay on its side, was seized with diarrhoea, vomited blood and died in twenty-five minutes.[1]

Portier and Richet named the new phenomenon anaphylaxis, from the Greek roots *phylaxis*, meaning "protection,"

and *ana* meaning "the opposite of." This contrasted with pro-
phylaxis, the giving of vaccine injections for protection.
Within a year Arthus had shown that the same anaphylaxis
could be caused by substances which were otherwise quite
bland and harmless if there were repeated injections. Nowadays we know that the irritating effects of insect bites are
more often caused by our own earlier sensitisation to the
antigens in the saliva of the insects than by any poison injected by such harmless creatures as gnats.

Right from the start it was held, notably by Arthus, that
anaphylaxis was an immunological phenomenon. The point
was not only proved to be true, but shown to be useful almost immediately. Those were the high days of serum therapy, the first decade of the twentieth century, when it was
realised that by following in the footsteps of Pasteur the infectious diseases could be beaten; when typhoid had first
been controlled among the British troops in the Boer War;
and when some enthusiasts prophesied extraordinary triumphs for serotherapy in all sorts of conditions, claims
which we can now see to have been unjustified. The great
problem of serotherapy was that repeated injections with
serum could give rise to anaphylactic shock and death, or to
the slower, more delayed onset of symptoms of serum sickness. The problem has not been completely solved to this
day, and it took thirty years to achieve any great ameliora-
tion. But nowadays we can treat serum prepared in some
other species of animal (often the horse) with enzymes
which have a fairly mild digestive action so that the antibody-carrying immunoglobulins manufactured by the horse
retain their protective activity against infectious organisms
but lose most of their antigenicity and therefore their power
to provoke immune reactions in us.

The connection between anaphylaxis, serum sickness,
and immunology was virtually established as early as 1905

by the Austrians von Pirquet and Schick, though the big
theoretical difficulty in proving the case was that in some in-
stances an animal sensitised so as to undergo anaphylactic
shock could not be shown to have specific antibody in its circulation. But von Pirquet had an even more profound effect
on the development of the ideas of immunology.

First and foremost he demolished, by experiment and argument, the "teleological" notion that antibodies were designed as a specific mechanism to defend the body from invasion. Von Pirquet proposed instead that the immune system
should be regarded as a whole, and that its reaction to antigens varied according to the particular circumstances. According to his view, and it is one we now accept, the arrival
of an antigen causes different states of reactivity. A major
factor deciding the reactivity of the immune system to the
presence of an antigen is whether it has met that antigen
before. But previous sensitisation does not, in principle,
change the fact that the immune system can react in three
different ways upon the arrival of antigen:

1. The immune system can be paralysed; the obvious examples of this are tolerance and immunological deficiency.
2. Defensive immune reactions, such as we have so far considered normal and advantageous, take place and these reactions will differ in speed according to whether or not there
has been previous sensitisation or immunisation.
3. Various hypersensitive reactions take place.

Von Pirquet did not know about the role of lymphocytes or
the cooperating two-armed mechanism of the immune system; but his appreciation of the varied reactivity of the system, sometimes favorable, sometimes not, at the approach of
antigen is one of the foundations of the modern approach.

He was also the man who coined the term "allergy." We
do not use the word nowadays in the way he proposed. But

"allergy" is used to describe many forms of hypersensitive reaction. Most forms of hay fever and asthma are allergies —allergic reactions to pollen dust from the blooming flowers of early summer or to house dust which contains mites and the organic remains of other tiny creatures. And, even if we do not suffer from it ourselves, we have all met people who have violent allergic reactions to certain forms of food—not just the slightly exotic allergies to shellfish or strawberries. There are also people who suffer from "milk intolerance," and a few rare individuals can be found who are allergic to very many ordinary foods such as eggs and fish. It is quite common to find people who are allergic to certain drugs; penicillin is a well-known example. (A word or two of caution, though; allergies to drugs may not always be true immunological allergies. It is quite possible that in some cases of people who are "sensitive to penicillin" there may be an obscure metabolic difference, perhaps some unknown inability to manufacture a particular enzyme, which causes the drug to produce anomalous results.)

Nowadays it is possible, and indeed quite common, to be treated for allergies if they are of a disabling sort, such as intolerance to an ordinary foodstuff like eggs. In simple terms the treatment is to inject the patient many times with small doses of purified extracts of the substance to which he is allergic. Each injection raises a red weal at the site on the skin, but eventually the unwanted immune reaction to the substance is apparently paralysed and the patient can face bacon and eggs at breakfast as well as anyone. It is not really known how this treatment works, but the results are usually satisfactory as long as the particular substance which rouses the allergic reaction can be identified. The problem with hay fever and asthma is that there are so many different pollens in the air, so many types of organic remains in the house dust, that the precise substance which precipitates an attack in the case of any one of innumerable sufferers can rarely be established, and then only after a long and tedious process of elimination.

Discussing allergies has led me too far ahead of my story. The study of hypersensitivities was one of the principal interests of immunological researchers in the years around the First World War. It was soon established that hypersensitivity could be transferred "passively" from one animal to another, in the same way that the early students of immunity showed that they could transfer protection against infectious bacteria from one animal to another. Then, in 1921, work which was primarily directed against tuberculosis showed that there was another type of hypersensitivity: a kind which only revealed itself several hours or even days after the antigen had been introduced into a sensitised body. This was given the obvious, though clumsy, name "delayed-type hypersensitivity."

It soon became clear that the two types of hypersensitivity differed not only in the time they needed to manifest themselves, but also in something more fundamental. Ordinary hypersensitivity, and its extreme form of anaphylactic shock and death, could only be transferred from one animal to another by blood serum; delayed hypersensitivity, which can likewise cause death in extreme cases, could only be transferred from one animal to another by the transfer of whole cells. As is so often the case, later experiments have compelled us to admit that there is a spectrum of effects rather than a clear-cut difference, a spectrum both in the time taken to manifest hypersensitivity and in the comparative abundance of antibody and activated cells in the reaction. But the broad conclusion is clear. Here is strong supportive evidence for the idea that the immune system is a two-part system, with an antibody side and a cell-mediated side. Immediate hypersensitivity is a reaction of circulating blood-born antibody; delayed hypersensitivity is a cell-mediated reaction. It can even be shown that lymphocytes are probably the most important type of cells in transferring delayed hypersensitivity.

Probably the most widely known example of cell-mediated delayed hypersensitivity is the Mantoux skin test for tuberculosis. An injection of tuberculin (a filtrate of tubercle bacilli containing proteins from the bacillus) produces no effect on a person who has never contracted TB. But in the case of a patient who has got tuberculosis it produces a small red lump on the skin at the site of the injection. The lump begins to form some hours after the injection has been given and reaches its final size as much as forty-eight hours later. Apart from the time it takes to develop there is little difference between the outward appearance of a positive reaction to the Mantoux test and the red weal produced at the site of an injection of egg, milk, or fish protein during tests for allergies. But close examination of the two marks shows that the allergic weal is filled with liquid, while the Mantoux test reaction contains a solid mass of cells, mostly macrophages and lymphocytes. (Let me re-emphasise here that allergic and delayed-hypersensitivity reactions can be precipitated by antigens in any form, either by proteins alone or by cell-carried antigens in the form of invasive bacteria or transplanted tissues; it is only in *transferring* sensitivity from one animal to another that the difference between serum-transferred immediate hypersensitivity and cell-transferred delayed hypersensitivity can be observed.)

But the Mantoux test to discover whether a patient was suffering from TB or not was in regular use for many years before Landsteiner and Chase finally proved that delayed hypersensitivity could be transferred from one animal to another, and that lymphocytes seemed to be the most active cells involved in this transfer. The work of Landsteiner and Chase was carried out in the United States in 1942. They rendered guinea-pigs hypersensitive to a simple chemical, picryl chloride, by painting the chemical onto the skin; this sensitivity could be transferred to other guinea-pigs only by the transfer of cells from the sensitised animal, not by the transfer of serum. Chase went on to show that his cell-transferable hypersensitivity was the same mechanism as that observed in the tuberculosis work which had always been known up to that time as bacterial allergy. And it was Chase who coined the term "delayed hypersensitivity."

There is a slightly malicious story often told by immunologists about the discovery of delayed hypersensitivity; I have never been able to find out whether or not it is true. Landsteiner was awarded a Nobel Prize for this work with Chase. It was Landsteiner's second Nobel award, his first having been given forty years before for his discovery in his native Europe of the ABO blood groups, in 1900. The story is that Landsteiner really considered the experiment, of trying to transfer the picryl chloride sensitivity of one set of guinea-pigs to another by cell transfer, useless and a waste of perfectly good laboratory guinea-pigs. Chase is alleged to have done the work while Landsteiner was away on holiday and presented the old man with the striking results when he returned to the laboratories. However, since Landsteiner was also the pioneer of the work with haptens as immunological agents, and since he did not receive a Nobel award for this or for his work with viruses, perhaps justice has been done, whatever the truth about the discovery of delayed hypersensitivity.

The other commonly known form of delayed hypersensitivity, which in principle was revealed in the nature of the discovery of the phenomenon, is contact dermatitis. Most forms of industrial dermatitis (skin rashes and skin disease caused by constant contact with organic material in factory processes) fall into this category.

By treating allergies and hypersensitivity after discussing

the main theories of the science of self, and by referring to the fact that they give supportive evidence to the main theories, I have perhaps done them less than justice. The discoveries of the phenomena, and much of the research into them, happened before the development of the main theories. At several times they were the most exciting topics of research in immunology. And the fact of the matter is that the main theories of the science of self arose as much from the study of hypersensitivity as from the study of infectious disease and the immune reactions against it.

But having now brought the story of hypersensitivity into line with the other immune responses such as tolerance and the normal defensive reaction, we must ask two important questions: How does the hypersensitive response differ from the other responses? And why should there be such a response at all? There are no very clear answers to these questions.

The sequence of events that leads to hypersensitive reaction we assume to start in exactly the same way as that leading to other responses. An antigen enters the body: it may react immediately with circulating antibody that is specific to it, if it has been there before; it will meet lymphocytes carrying the specific antibody. The lymphocytes are triggered off into reaction and at this point the hypersensitive reaction differs from the other reactions. Here is the main gap in our knowledge, a blank space that stretches out on the map until we come to the final stages in the reaction, which indicates two really important differences between the hypersensitive reaction and other immune reactions.

In cases of immediate hypersensitivity, or allergies, a different type of antibody, the IgE antibody, is produced. This IgE never seems to be produced in large quantities; consequently, it has not been very well studied. But in hypersensitive reactions IgE is definitely produced, and when, probably along with other types of antibody, it gets into the circulation, it reacts with mast cells. These mast cells are large, specialised cells found in most parts of the body. The IgE attaches itself to the mast cells. Probably again acting in conjunction with other types of antibody and with complement, it breaks them open and releases their contents.

The peculiarity of mast cells—and therefore presumably their specialised purpose, although there are a number of unsolved questions about them—is that they contain large quantities of histamine and other powerful chemical substances normally found in the inflammation processes that follow any sort of wounding of body tissues. It is the release of histamine and its associated chemicals which causes the typical inflammatory symptoms of allergy.

In the case of delayed hypersensitivity, the most striking "differential" feature is again found in the final phases of the reaction. This is the appearance of lymphocytes which appear to be capable of killing other cells by their own actions. They are then called cytotoxic lymphocytes—"cytotoxic" meaning dangerous to other cells. In the other immune reactions lymphocytes are not observed in a killing role—they recognise antigen, they react to it, they proliferate, they develop into plasma cells producing specific antibody, and they probably cooperate with macrophages in using antibody to kill invading cells. But they do not appear to do the killing themselves except in delayed hypersensitive reactions. It is still an open question whether those lymphocytes which can be seen to invade transplanted tissue act in a cytotoxic role.

Why should there be hypersensitive reactions at all? This second question can be rephrased as, What is the biological meaning of this apparently disadvantageous variation of the immune system? One possible answer is that hypersensitivity is simply an inherent part of a mechanism we do not fully understand and that its disadvantages are comparatively so slight that it has not, in evolutionary terms, been worth getting rid of. But a rather more constructive answer can be suggested in terms of the science of self.

There are hints, not much more, that the hypersensitive reactions may have had a role specifically in defense against internal parasites. It seems that IgE may be particularly effective in causing reactions of an inflammatory type in the tiny folds of the intestine, that is, in those places where worms (technically, helminths) desire to attach themselves. IgE appears to be present in larger quantities than usual in cases of patients infected with worms. A similar slight hint comes in the field of delayed hypersensitivity—notably, in the case of the hydatid worms, which seem to produce a distinct, specific delayed hypersensitivity response. This is used clinically as the standard test for discovering whether a patient has an infection of this type of worm. And although such a test (similar to the Mantoux test) is not the method of choice, in other cases it is known that types of worm and protozoal infections do produce specific delayed hypersensitivities. At the same time inhaled pollen grains also appear to cause the manufacture of larger-than-usual quantities of IgE.

The more closely we look at delayed hypersensitivity the more advantageous it seems, despite the discomfort and disability it produces in forms like dermatitis. There are, for instance, the very interesting results of McKinness, who immunised animals with brucella organisms (brucella causes the disease of spontaneous abortion in cattle and can affect man, sometimes fatally). He found that in the immunised animals the macrophages had increased power to kill brucella organisms when a challenge dose of these organisms was introduced. But there was no serum factor present—no detectable anti-brucella antibody. The resistance to the organism must therefore have been of the cell-transferable type, and the "immunity" was a delayed hypersensitive reaction. The Mantoux test for the presence of immune reaction against tubercle bacilli also shows that an "immunity" (a defensive reaction) can be based on cell-mediated, delayed hypersensitivity rather than on the more usual antibody base. Similar results can be shown in the case of many fungal infections and with the comparatively common "salmonella" organisms—the causes of paratyphoid and forms of food-poisoning. We just do not know why some infective organisms should elicit a cell-mediated immunity rather than an antibody-based reaction.

It is reasonable to speculate, however, that one of the importances of the cell-mediated response might be as a countermeasure to virus infection. Viruses grow and multiply within cells; they must be right inside the cell in order to use its own machinery to manufacture replicas of themselves. Only when the virus has multiplied so much that it kills the host cell is it released into the blood stream, and to the rest of the body where antibody molecules can get at it. Antibody molecules cannot get into the cell where the virus is multiplying. There is thus an obvious advantage to be gained by having a system in which cytotoxic lymphocytes could attack cells where the virus-multiplication process is going on. But we have no proof that this does happen nor do we know that a cell containing multiplying virus shows any external, virus-revealing antigens—except in the case of those cells which have been transformed by virus into cancer cells.

When we come to the cell-mediated response to the body's own cells which have been transformed into cancer cells (whether that transformation has come about by chance variation or by chemical or viral action), we can see no appreciable difference between the cell-mediated, delayed hypersensitive reaction and the cell-mediated response of the immunological surveillance system. It is very significant that the operation of "neo-natal thymectomy"—the removal of the thymus of an animal immediately after birth which was such an important experimental method for clinching the argument about the main features of the immune system—reduces not only the resistance to transplants but also the delayed hypersensitivity responses of the animal.

Nevertheless, there is considerably more hope now for sufferers from allergic reactions than there was even when I started writing this book; 1970 has seen a number of really important steps forward in the field. In particular, the mode of action of the antibody peculiar to allergic reactions, the IgE immunoglobulin, has been made much clearer.

The essence of an immediate allergic reaction is the production of this particular antibody, IgE, in response to the arrival of a specific antigen, and the migration of the IgE onto mast cells. The mast cells are then attacked by the IgE and their contents of inflammatory chemicals such as histamine released, causing the weals and eruptions typical of allergy. What has now been made clear is that it is the combination of antibody and antigen which fixes itself onto the mast cells. Even more fascinating and thought-provoking is the conclusion that the IgE/antigen combination does not break open the mast cell ("lysis," which is what had been thought to happen). Instead, the combination allows or encourages the inflammatory chemicals to be released through the wall of the mast cell without breaking the wall. It also seems highly likely that IgG antibody, probably specific against the same antigen, cooperates in this process in some way.

The transport of important chemical substances through the cell wall is believed to be quite a common feature of the functions of living bodies. It is, for instance, likely that insulin and the hormones have to be transported through the cell wall when they reach their target cells, although there are theories that the arrival of the hormones on the outside surface of the target cells is enough to signal the start of the appropriate activities inside. So there is possible doubt whether such important substances actually penetrate cells from outside. Certainly these hormones—and also the antibodies which figure so prominently in immunology—are manufactured inside cells and released to the rest of the body. And it is believed that enzymes are responsible for most if not all transport of substances through cell walls, though in the case of allergic reactions there is no firm knowledge of what enzymes are involved or how they work.

The important point is that the greater knowledge of the action of IgE on mast cells, even though we do not know all the details of the interaction, opens up a much wider variety of possibilities of checking the action. At the moment treatment for allergies tends to concentrate on the peripheries of the process. We can desensitise some allergic patients by injections which "overwhelm" or "paralyse" the unwanted immune response, but finding out exactly what foreign proteins are causing the allergy can be a tedious business. Or we can deal with the symptom of the allergic reaction as we treat asthma, by giving bronchodilatory drugs—drugs which chemically relax and dilate the bronchial tree in direct opposition to the immune reaction which is tightening up the air passages. Or we give antihistamines to try to neutralise the output of the mast cells.

The new knowledge of the processes involved in the IgE/mast cell reaction gives us other links in the chain which we could try to break. We could attempt to reduce the production of IgG if it is shown to be cooperating in the IgE/mast cell reaction. We could try to block the mast cell receptors to which the IgE attaches. We could try to occupy and fill up the antibody-binding sites on the IgE with some substance other than the antigen, so that the IgE/antigen combination cannot perform its work of exciting and allowing the release of mast cell contents.

But the link in the chain that seems most prone to attack is the point at which the enzymes transport the histamines and other inflammatory chemicals across the cell wall. The possibilities of inhibiting either the enzyme formation or activity appear considerable. One drug has already been found which seems effective against many allergic reactions; no one knows quite how it works but there are suspicions that it blocks a receptor site at some part of the process.

One reason for predicting that considerable progress will soon be achieved in dealing with at least the simpler, antibody-induced allergies (as opposed to the more complicated cell-mediated hypersensitivities) is precisely that the pharmaceutical companies have considerable financial incentive to produce drugs which will interfere with this immune reaction. It is symptomatic that immunological departments have been set up by a number of pharmaceutical research establishments recently and that the field of allergy is one of their chief studies.

It looks, then, as if we must regard allergic reactions as being as much part of the immune system as any other reaction. In some respects they certainly are different, and many of them are characterised by a much more speedy reactivity. At least some are plainly advantageous, and many more may be so, in fact or at least in origin. I am sorry for the sufferers from hay fever; I am sorry for myself when I have it. But it looks as though it is an inseparable part of being oneself and able to recognise the fact.

Auto-Immunity

Auto-immunity is quite different from allergy in the respect that it definitely means something has gone wrong. It is a disease state. The mechanisms involved in the auto-immune diseases, however, and many of the obvious symptoms, are the same as those in allergies. It is fashionable now, and possibly more correct, to refer to these disease states as "auto-allergic" diseases. I shall continue, nevertheless, to call them auto-immune diseases, because I think this makes the distinction clear.

Auto-immunity means that a body launches immune reactions against parts of itself. Antibody is manufactured against the antigens appearing on the body's own cells, just as if those antigens belonged to some other individual. Auto-immunity is thus the treatment of self as if it were not-self. The fact that, in certain types of disease where there is no other visible causative organism, auto-antibodies can be found, is a support for the main theories of the science of the self, since in non-disease states it is impossible to find auto-antibodies.

But note that I have been careful to avoid saying that the manufacture of auto-antibodies *causes* these disease states. Such caution is symptomatic of the present state of opinion about auto-immune diseases generally, a state of confusion and conflicting views. Auto-immunity seemed such a clear light when it was first discovered. It confirmed the shining new theories of the science of self. It seemed to offer such prospects for progress against a number of conditions that had hitherto proved intractable largely because they lacked any obvious cause. The theory of auto-immunity still stands, the discoveries confirm the self/not-self approach to immunity; but as we approach each separate "auto-immune disease," the concept seems to blur at the edges and escape our grasp.

The possibility that auto-immunity might occur as a catastrophe had been foreseen, or at least imagined, by that extraordinary pioneer of immunology Ehrlich as early as 1901:

The organism possesses certain contrivances by means of which the immunity reaction, so easily produced by all kinds of cells, is prevented from acting against the organism's own elements and so giving rise to autotoxins. Further investigations made by us have confirmed this view, so that one might be justified in speaking of a "horror autotoxicus" of the organism. These contrivances are naturally of the highest importance for the existence of the individual.[2]

In the same work he says, "Only when the internal regulating contrivances are no longer intact can great dangers arise." Sixty-nine years later, Professor J. V. Dacie, of the Royal Postgraduate Medical School, London, added the comment: "The concept of 'horror autotoxicus' still stands, and even if the internal regulating contrivances are still largely unknown, the suggestion that their breakdown could lead to great dangers still holds."

Auto-antibodies were first observed in the 1930's, under very peculiar experimental circumstances. There are some tissues of the body that do appear to have antigens that are quite specific to themselves: some eye-lens tissue, the cells that form male sperm, and the myelinated cells of the brain. All these tissues are normally separated from the rest of the body by special barriers which keep out the circulating blood. Yet when experimental animals were injected with these tissues from other animals of the same species they made antibodies against them, and these antibodies could be shown to react against the same corresponding tissues in themselves. But the antibodies, the auto-antibodies, were not apparently harmful; they were not found in disease states, only under these rather "forced" experimental conditions—so they seemed irrelevant to human clinical disease.

Then in 1945 Coombs, Mourant, and Race discovered auto-antibodies attached to red cells and apparently destroying them in an obscure form of human anaemia. Within a year

Boorman showed that there was a positive Coombs test (i.e., there were auto-antibodies) in patients who developed this type of anaemia late in life, but not in patients who developed it congenitally or through heredity. This particular anaemia is called haemolytic anaemia—"haemolytic" meaning that the red cells are being destroyed. Yet, oddly enough, no one seems to have recognised this as what we now call auto-immune disease. The only reasonable explanation of this is the fascinating thought that there was at that time no theoretical structure which provided a place for auto-immune disease; Ehrlich had been virtually forgotten and the science of self had not yet been conceived. This is one of the strongest pieces of evidence for the importance of Burnet's science of self concept: a whole block of existing medical evidence suddenly found a meaning when his theories were widely grasped.

As we have seen, in the very early 1950's Burnet's theories were suddenly given life by the demonstration that tolerance existed and could be obtained artificially. But a body, unless it is persuaded in its earliest stages that some not-self tissues are really self, will normally react against any not-self antigen. The question remains as to how an immune system "knows" what is self. We believe that the body produces lymphocytes equipped to recognise all possible antigens. There is no obvious reason why it should not produce lymphocytes equipped to react against its own self antigens. The obvious explanation, though it has not been proved, is that each one of us is in fact "tolerant" to ourselves. In the early stages of the development of the immune system, just before and immediately after birth, the anti-self lymphocytes which are produced are presumably overwhelmed by the vast abundance of self antigen. The whole system of reaction against self is paralysed by the enormous amount of self antigen that is present—in just the same way as enormous doses of foreign antigen can paralyse the immune system of an adult animal in experimental conditions. Furthermore, tolerance, as achieved by the Medawar method, can only be maintained by the continued presence of the foreign antigen. In the case of our own bodies, we keep those lines of lymphocytes which could react against ourselves paralysed by the enormous doses of self antigen which we naturally possess. (Or perhaps the original anti-self lymphocytes are killed by the massiveness of the dose of self antigen before they can proliferate, and all subsequent productions of the same type are likewise killed.)

Once this view of the nature of immunity and self-tolerance had been put forward and, to some extent, established, it became clear that the immune system could theoretically break down and allow the production of auto-antibodies. Any breakdown of this sort must be auto-aggressive. Within a couple of years of the publication of the work of Medawar, Billingham, and Brent the existence of auto-immune disease had, indeed, been established. But it was not haemolytic anaemia that provided the proof, it was a rather rare thyroid disease called Hashimoto's disease.

In America E. Witebsky and N. Rose demonstrated, in 1956, that if they injected rabbits with thyroglobulin from other rabbits mixed with a suitable adjuvant (or "helper" in immunological terms), their animals would suffer a short-lived inflammation of the thyroid and could be shown to be making antibodies against their own thyroglobulin. The thyroid is the gland at the base of the neck whose major activity seems to be regulating the speed at which the body's chemistry works. Its product is chiefly thyroglobulin and, broadly speaking, the more of this the thyroid produces the more active the person. Correspondingly, if the thyroid does not produce enough thyroglobulin people become sluggish. But the experiment of Witebsky and Rose could be compared to the experiments of the 1930's mentioned above because normally thyroglobulin does not reach the circulation and is both produced in and retained by the thyroid. Rose himself later proved that this was not the case; but in the meantime this American work had provided the vital stimulus to the work of Ivan Roitt and Deborah Doniach at the Middlesex Hospital in London.

Ivan Roitt had been pondering the problem of cancer and immunity. He was working on the problems of tumours producing their own antigens, and wondered why the body's normal immune reactions might not be provoked against these antigens. Deborah Doniach was working in the same hospital but rather closer to the clinical side. She was the one actually studying Hashimoto's disease and had been looking at the gammaglobulins present in people suffering from it. In particular, she had noticed that there were a great many plasma cells producing antibodies in the thyroid of people suffering from the disease. The idea that Hashimoto's disease might be an auto-immune disease, a case of the body attacking its own constituents, arose in talk between the two researchers, both of whom had read a brief abstract of the work of Witebsky and Rose. Once this had taken shape in their minds, it was only a question of performing a comparatively simple test. There were no long months of patient testing of specially bred laboratory mice. In Roitt's own words, "We set it all up in a few days. We simply shovelled together the patients' extracts and their serum and waited for the precipitations."

In other words, they took thyroid tissue from the patients with Hashimoto's disease. They put it together with their blood serum, each patient's thyroid tissue matched against his own gammaglobulins, and waited to see whether there was the familiar visible precipitation of particles which would show that antibodies in the blood serum were binding together with constituents of the patients' own thyroid glands. The answers were clear. Patients with Hashimoto's disease made auto-antibodies, antibodies which attacked their own thyroid tissue.

Once a clear case of auto-immune disease had been established, the hunt was on. People began to look for signs of auto-immunity in almost every disease where the cause was unknown; and very rapidly they found it. Auto-antibodies turned up in systemic lupus erythematosus, nephrosis, multiple sclerosis, Addison's disease, ulcerative colitis, and chronic active liver disease. Add to the list the haemolytic anaemia in which auto-antibodies had first been found, and also pernicious anaemia. Most exciting of all, because the diseases are so common and so painful, auto-antibodies could be shown to exist in rheumatoid arthritis and rheumatic fever. And, by now, even cases of cell-mediated immune reactions against self-tissue can be demonstrated.

The excitement, naturally enough, was fairly intense in the early 1960's. Here, in auto-immunity, we had an explanation for a wide variety of previously puzzling diseases, diseases, what is more, of such varied type, affecting the skin, the joints and connective tissue, the liver, the kidneys, the blood, and glands like the thyroid and the adrenals. Obviously, if we could suppress or change this auto-immune response, we might be able to treat this wide variety of diseases.

But, frankly, once the identification of auto-immune processes in these diseases had been made, remarkably little progress followed. Though a large amount of work continues in the field, the excitement and the hope of dramatic clinical results has now largely evaporated.

The real problem is the failure to prove that it is an auto-immune reaction which *causes* these diseases. It now appears likely in more and more cases that the auto-immune reaction may only be a consequence of some other disease process. Take the case of ulcerative colitis, a by no means rare disease of the intestines. Auto-antibodies can clearly be shown here but it is considered probable that this is simply a cross-reaction to the presence of gut-bacteria antigens. Cross-reaction between antibody and antigen for which it is not specific is only to be expected—after all, antibody is basically only a shape to fit another shape, the shape of antigen. Sometimes, by chance, shapes will be similar, and some shapes will always be more alike than others. So in ulcerative colitis it has been suggested that the body mounts a normal response to certain bacteria present in the gut, and the antibody produced in this response is of such a shape and nature that it attacks the gut as well. Since normally we tolerate a wide variety of useful or harmless bacteria in our gut, the cause of these cases of auto-immune ulcerative colitis is therefore the abnormal reaction to the gut bacteria rather than the auto-immune phenomenon.

Similarly, in many of the other cases of auto-immune disease there is now scientific controversy over whether the aetiology (the essential causative machinery) is auto-immunity or whether the auto-immune reaction is an epiphenomenon, something that appears in the course of events but is non-causative.

Not surprisingly, perhaps, the two diseases which still seem most likely to be *caused* by auto-immune reactions are thyroiditis and haemolytic anaemia. Earlier in this chapter I quoted Professor J. V. Dacie. In the Kettle Memorial Lecture delivered to the Royal College of Pathologists in London in February 1970, entitled "Auto-immune Haemolytic Anaemias," Dacie said, "It has to be admitted that the problem of why an individual, after perhaps many years of apparently good health, starts to form antibodies against antigens on his red cells that he has previously tolerated is still largely unsolved. In all probability there is no single or simple explanation."

There are no fewer than four possible explanations that we can see at the moment, and there is really very little evidence in favour of any of them. It could well be that the antigens on the red cells are changed in some way. The action of a virus, or a body chemical like an enzyme, or of some chemical that the body has taken in, such as a drug, could cause this change of antigen in theory. Once the antigen on the red cells has changed to a form previously not encountered by the body, the red cells will be treated as foreign and antibodies against them will be formed. A second possibility could be the cross-reaction situation similar to the explanation of ulcerative colitis given above. In this case the antigen against which the antibody has been formed could be anything under the sun, though some invading virus or bacteria is obviously the most likely. And if cross-reaction is the cause, if it really is a case of properly formed antibody against some invader attacking the body cells by sheer chance likeness of shape, then this is a case of rotten bad luck for the individual to whom it happens. Yet another alternative is that for some reason the body suddenly increases its ability to manufacture antibodies. This sudden stepping-up of the antibody-manufacturing process might conceivably lead to the production of auto-antibodies as well as larger quantities of the natural defensive antibody. Finally, there is the original, pure science of self explanation—that there arises a "forbidden" clone of anti-self lymphocytes, forbidden but not malignant. This means a breakdown of self-tolerance, either because of the unexplained persistence of some cells which should have been eliminated in early life, or because of the failure of the normal immune processes which paralyse or eliminate such forbidden cells when they arise. This is the pure auto-immune disease.

At the moment we lack the evidence to decide between the four explanations or whether any of them is correct. Even if we could establish that some disease quite definitely had an auto-immune aetiology, there would be the problem of how to treat it. Plain immuno suppression, using the same techniques as are used in preventing transplant rejection, would obviously reduce the production of auto-antibodies. But, as we know in the case of transplants, it would also reduce the effectiveness of the body's defences against a host of everyday viruses, bacteria, and fungi. And what good would immuno suppression do? Presumably as soon as the drug regime ended, the production of auto-antibodies would start again. Direct treatment of the inflammatory symptoms which are usually the result of auto-immune reactions is quite possible using the steroids (cortisone, etc.). But this seems to offer no more than a palliation of symptoms—as in the case of cortisone treatment of rheumatism—and cannot be continued for too long with such potent chemicals.

Only a direct attack on the lymphocytes appears to offer much of a long-term solution. But there seems no way at the moment of selecting those families of lymphocytes which are doing the damage and sparing the remaining families whose presence we need.

The immunologists have, if the truth be told, run out of ideas for ways to attack auto-immune phenomena, irrespective of whether these reactions are truly causative or only the result of some other predisposing pathogenesis.

A third cause for gloom is the lack of hope of any useful clinical outcome in the immediate future. This is because of the growing body of evidence that the actual tissue damage in cases of auto-immune disease—the damage to cartilage and bone surface in cases of rheumatoid arthritis, for instance—may be caused by antibody-antigen complexes rather than by the auto-antibodies themselves. In these complexes the antibody binds onto the antigen in the way it is supposed to do. But apparently, instead of being swept up and removed or digested by the macrophages, the lump of antibody and antigen remains in the tissues and, certainly in the case of rheumatoid arthritis, seems to form a focus of inflammation.

Antibody-antigen complexes can also be found in the inflammations produced in some cases of hypersensitivity or allergy, especially when the more usual types of immunoglobulin accompany IgE in the breaking open of mast cells. This has led to the suspicion that there may be some relationship, at least in terms of the mechanism involved, between the inflammations of hypersensitivity and of autoimmunity. And just as one can consider the hypersensitivities as examples of changed reactivity in the immune system, it is not unreasonable to regard auto-immunities as yet another type of changed reactivity. It is for reasons such as these that some scientists have favored changing the name "auto-immunity" to "auto-allergy," and prefer the term "auto-allergic diseases" for the group of diseases in which auto-antibodies appear. This very neatly brings the meaning of "allergy" back to almost exactly what its originator, von Pirquet, proposed. But apart from this slight historical satisfaction there is little else in the story of auto-immune diseases which would bring any sort of intellectual pleasure at the moment.

The very latest developments, far from proffering much hope of clarifying the problems, seem instead to suggest even more confusion. A number of research groups on both sides of the Atlantic have noticed recently some prevalence of auto-immune types of disease among sufferers from diabetes. In July 1970, a group in Edinburgh provided firm confirmation of this in a large study of more than 1,000 diabetics. They found that diabetics were in fact more likely to have

auto-immune diseases than non-diabetic controls. Furthermore, they found auto-antibodies against thyroid and gut
cells in diabetics who had no clinical signs of thyroid or
other auto-immune disease. For some quite unknown reason
these tendencies to auto-immune reactions seem to be more
pronounced in diabetics who are dependent on insulin. But
the meaning of this relationship between diabetes and auto-
immunity is quite obscure, because plainly auto-immunity
can exist independently of diabetes.

The analogy between the immune system and a police
force seems helpful once again in explaining the confusion
that reigns in this field. The case is one of subversion within
the force. Instead of confining itself to dealing with criminals
and spies, the police have suddenly taken to attacking perfectly loyal and honest citizens—and this not at the behest of
a dictator who has gained control of the force, but apparently against the general interest of the community, perhaps
at the suggestion of some foreign power.

Well, who can police the police? Who can investigate the
investigators? Where would one start to root out such subversion? Under these circumstances the rulers of the community would be unable to trust any police officer even to con-
duct the enquiry into the root cause of the subversion. And
any attempt to get rid of the subversive policemen might be
thwarted by the subversive forces themselves.

Unless one can find out the origin of the subversion it is
impossible to reform the police force. The only alternative
seems to be to dismiss every single policeman and start off
again with a fresh lot. Apart from the problem of doing this
at all, and the complete lack of a police force while it is happening, there may well be appalling injustice done to the
loyal and honest officers in the disgraced force. And who will
train and organise the new police force to be recruited?

There are obvious exaggerations and dangers in equating

live policemen with lymphocytes, but the analogy may at least enlist our sympathies for the scientists who are trying to unravel the tremendous problems of auto-immunity.

Chapter 10

The Failures of Immunology

The Common Cold

"Scientists! They can't even cure the common cold." This is the classic gibe against science today. You can hear it said in every tone from the sneer of that anti-intellectualism which I find one of the most disturbing features of Western society at the present time to the happy insouciance of the man at the bar or the taxi driver. Pronounced in more solemn tones, it can also be heard from the younger side of the generation gap, along with a condemnation of scientists and their technologies as the producers of the atom bomb and pollution. The whole blame for this failure cannot be laid on the shoulders of the immunologists; presumably the chemists and biologists of the drug-manufacturing industry have also failed to produce an answer to the common cold. But there is no doubt that the science of immunology has attacked the problem of the common cold and been baffled by it. And the reason for this failure is a fascinating one—it is that the cause of the common cold is too "common" to be treated by the methods of immunology on any practical basis.

It is poetic justice that England, famed for its cold, damp, and variable weather, should have provided the leading assault on the problem of the common cold and also should have been the place where it was shown why the problem is so intractable. It all began just after the end of the Second World War with a gesture of American generosity.

The Harvard Hospital, headquarters of the Medical Research Council Common Cold Research Unit, is a collection of well-built and well-equipped wooden buildings grouped round a central administrative block on the downland just above Salisbury, the cathedral city which is the county town of Wiltshire and one of the most attractive places in Britain. It had been built and largely staffed by Harvard as an American laboratory and hospital during the years of the war; when hostilities ended it was offered, lock, stock, and barrel, to the British government.

The man who transformed it into a common cold research unit was Sir Christopher Andrewes, who had been closely involved in the influenza research of the 1930's at the Medical Research Council's Hampstead laboratories. His initiative and his administrative effort brought about the start of the new unit. But it was a combination of the physical shape of the war-time hospital and the nature of the scientific problems involved in studying the common cold that dictated the unusual course of the research that followed.

Up to then no one had isolated a causative organism for the common cold. Even more difficult, from the scientific point of view, was the fact that there was no "animal model system"—in other words, no one could show that any laboratory animal suffered from the common cold or could be made to suffer from it. It is very rarely realised that in the majority of cases of infectious diseases the crucial step leading to the conquest of the disease has been the discovery of a way of infecting an animal species with the human disease. Indeed, this is the usual method of proving that a disease is caused by a transmissible organism, long before that organism has been identified and isolated. Again, it is usually by the study of experimentally infected animals that the precise mode of attack of the organism is elucidated, and very often the organism is finally isolated from animal tissues. The animal in which the disease can be established should be of such a size and nature that it can be kept and handled in fairly large numbers in the laboratory. It would really not be very useful to find that the common cold could be successfully transmitted to elephants and tigers. Correspondingly, one of the most important advances in recent years in the research on leprosy has been the discovery that the causative organism can be cultivated in the foot-pads of laboratory mice.

There was some earlier, rather doubtful evidence from the work of Kruse at the Hygienic Institute of the University of Leipzig in 1914 that a virus might be responsible for some colds. In 1923 Olitsky and MacCartney in New York first succeeded in giving colds to chimpanzees, though it was not scientifically established until 1931, when Dochez at the Presbyterian Hospital in New York, using a specially built up, carefully isolated group of eight chimpanzees, showed that they could be given colds from the filtrates of materials from human beings with colds. Furthermore, the chimpanzees were shown to be able to infect each other with colds by contact. The efforts to grow or "culture" the causative organism, though apparently successful in some cases in the New York laboratories, were not confirmed in other centres, however. In any case, chimpanzees are far too big and expensive to maintain as laboratory animals. And they tend to disturb the innocent virologists by apparently studying the doctors just as inquisitively as the latter study the apes.

This work lapsed after the early 1930's undoubtedly because of the great rush of progress in the study of influenza in the middle of that decade, after the successful demonstration of influenza in ferrets by the MRC workers at Hampstead. For those who like coincidences of the "small world" variety, Sir Christopher Andrewes claims that the virus which was used to infect the Hampstead ferrets came from no less a 'flu sufferer than himself. We must remember, too, that as recently as the 1930's there was no method of seeing or identifying a new virus, as no electron microscope existed. If tissue from an infected subject produced the same disease when injected into an experimental animal, then it was logical to assume that there was a causative, infectious organism involved. Bacteria could be isolated and seen under the microscope. But if the infected tissue was passed through a filter whose pores were so small that no bacteria could pass through, and it still caused infection, something smaller than a bacterium must cause the disease. Thus the very existence of virus was known only by its ability to cause disease—it was simply a "filterable agent," an organism small enough to pass through a filter, active enough to cause a disease, but never seen, never visualised, known only through its action.

So when work started at the Common Cold Research Unit at Salisbury the experimental animals had to be human volunteers. The production of a cold in an inoculated human being was the only real test available to the immunologists to show the presence of a cold virus. Sir Christopher Andrewes has since written: "As a method of work it was horribly clumsy, expensive and unreliable, but it was all we had." [1]

The great advantage of the war-time buildings up on the bleak but beautiful downland of Wiltshire (it is really part of Salisbury Plain, home of much of the British Army and of Stonehenge) was that it was easy to establish isolation from human contacts. The huts which had housed the American laboratory and hospital personnel were converted into living quarters for volunteers, connected only by long covered walkways. The volunteers, normally in pairs, were simply asked to come for ten days quiet holiday. Their rail fares were paid and they got a few shillings pocket-money a day. University students or teachers anxious to catch up on their reading were the most obvious source of volunteers—but it has been by no means unknown for impoverished couples to take their honeymoon as Common Cold volunteers. They are allowed to go for walks in the countryside as far as they wish; they must promise only to avoid the towns and approaching close to anyone they may meet. But many of the volunteers have so much enjoyed their ten days of peace and quiet that they have returned many times, the record for any one person being no fewer than twenty visits.

In the first three or four days of a visit virtually nothing happens. The idea is to weed out any volunteers who have arrived while actually incubating a cold caught outside the Unit. Then along comes the virologist with his experimental materials: either filtrates expected to produce a cold, because they are believed to contain virus, or harmless control materials, or materials which simply need to be investigated. The volunteers may be given the material by injection, by drops up the nose or in the eyes, by swabs on the throat, or by several other different methods. The common cold normally begins with a feeling of nasal congestion; it is very rarely accompanied by fever, and if fever does occur, it is slight. There is often a sore throat or similar symptom, but the classical feature is the large discharge of colourless mucous fluid from the nose; if this fluid turns yellow and thick, as it often does in the later stages of a cold, this is caused by secondary infection with other organisms. The most useful measurement of the severity of a cold established by the Salisbury researchers is the simple criterion of the number of paper handkerchiefs used by the sufferer.

Some volunteers accepted tougher treatment. They took hot baths and then stood about in draughty corridors for as much as a couple of hours. They sat about in wet clothes and wet socks. They allowed themselves to be chilled with fans. And the truth is that no one can prove that getting cold gives you a cold. In fact, colds are quite difficult to catch. But this book is about immunology and not about the common cold. And for fourteen years the Common Cold Research Unit just could not succeed in doing for the common cold what had been done for so many other infectious diseases.

Real progress, at least from an immunological point of view, did not come until the late 1950's. It came then principally because a new technique had been developed, the technique of tissue culture. Bacteria will grow in broth, in nutrient jellies on laboratory glass dishes, because they are creatures that can feed themselves in a way broadly analogous to how men feed themselves to survive and grow. Viruses do not feed; they enter a cell and take over the cell's mechanism to make it manufacture more of themselves. Viruses cannot grow or multiply outside cells. But cells or tissue taken from an adult animal will not normally survive for long when removed from their natural owner and placed in laboratory containers. Only tissue from embryos and from cancers can normally be persuaded to survive for many cell generations in the laboratory. (One of the most important technical advances of recent years has been the development by the American, Hayflick, of lines of non-cancerous human cells called diploid cells which can be kept alive and multiplying in the lab.) It was largely the work of Enders in Boston, mentioned earlier in connection with the development of polio vaccine, that made tissue culture in the laboratory a technique of enormous value in studying virus. Not the least significant feature of Enders's work was his demonstration that virus could be persuaded to grow in tissue cells of a type not normally associated with the attacks of the virus in disease; in other words, it was not necessary to have nose tissue in order to grow common cold virus.

By the middle 1950's the Common Cold Research Unit had established several "lines" of cold-causing material—but none of their attempts to grow an organism in the laboratory had succeeded. They could still only demonstrate the presence of an organism by causing human colds. Even when, for this reason, they believed they might be succeeding in growing cold virus in cultures, they could not prove it since they could find no trace of damage in the culture cells that might be caused by the growth of the virus. Then again came a new technique, this time called interference. The argument goes as follows. If you really do have a virus growing in infected tissue cultures, then when you put a second type of virus into that culture it ought to grow more slowly than if the culture were not infected, because the first virus is using up many of the cells for its own growth and these cells and their materials will not be available for the growth of the second virus. At Salisbury two viruses, named para-influenza 1 and ECHO 11, which are easily detectable by their ability to clump together red blood cells, were put into two sets of cultures, one suspected of containing cold virus and the other believed to be uninfected. Measured by the amount of red blood cells that were clumped, it was possible to show that the para-influenza and ECHO viruses both grew much more rapidly in uninfected cultures. Here at last was a method, albeit a rather complicated one, of showing that cold viruses could be obtained and grown in laboratory cultures.

The man who was largely responsible for this, and the immediately following successes, was D. A. J. Tyrrell, who is not an immunologist but a virologist. The work clearly is a modern replication in principle of the sort of thing that Pasteur and the great pioneers had done, and it is being repeated again at the present moment in the hunt for the organism that causes serum hepatitis.

The next improvement came from the decision to keep

the cultures rather cooler than the traditional temperature of body heat. Sure enough, the cold virus seemed to grow better at 33 degrees C. than at 37 degrees—not surprising in view of the fact that the virus inhabits the nose, where cold air from the outside world is warmed up to body temperature before being passed down to the lungs.

Then came a piece of luck. Something went wrong with the medium being used to surround the cells of the Salisbury culture tissue, and Tyrrell had to scrounge round other laboratories very quickly for fresh supplies of this standard medium. It was then noticed that in one of the cultures something strange was happening. It turned out that the borrowed medium was slightly more acid than the one originally used, and the slight acidity was so favourable to the cold virus that it was growing very rapidly and causing the culture tissue to degenerate. The ideal conditions for culture of the cold virus had been found and the clumsy interference tests could be dropped, too, because the virus was making its presence visible.

Normally in immunological history this is the stage at which the scientists can start considering the making of a protective vaccine. The agent has been found, it can be handled in the laboratory, it can be grown in culture so that by continual passagings from one culture to the next, it can be attenuated until it is harmless and usable as a vaccine. But with the common cold this was not to be the case.

The newly discovered and cultivated virus was shown to be a new type of organism (in 1960). It was named a rhinovirus (*rhino* from the Greek for "nose"). There were immediately hopes for the production of a vaccine, and industry was called in to help. But as the research went on, more and more different rhinoviruses were discovered. Then it was found that other viruses, which can cause other diseases, can also produce sometimes only the symptoms of the common cold:

para-influenza viruses, some of the ECHO viruses, some of the Coxsackie viruses, respiratory syncytial virus, and some of the entero viruses. There is no need to go into the nature and activities of all these; it is sufficient to say that at the moment more than one hundred different species, mostly rhinoviruses but also many other types, can cause the common cold.

In simple terms this means that there is virtually no hope of ever finding a vaccine against the common cold. The immunologists cannot prepare a vaccine against so many agents. They have been defeated by the sheer commonness of the common cold.

This is not the end of the story of the common cold. The disease still offers many problems to be solved, notably, why it occurs more often in winter; but it is the end for the moment as far as the immunologist is concerned.

Interferon

All is not lost in the battle against an infectious disease when the immunologists find they cannot make a suitable vaccine. For bacterial diseases there are the antibiotics. For virus diseases, however, the antibiotics have been little help so far. They cannot attack the virus multiplying inside cells for the most part, and there are precious few anti-viral drugs (possibly amantadine against 'flu and one chemical known to combat smallpox). Probably the greatest single hope of combating virus disease when it strikes those who have not been protected by vaccination is interferon. But it is still only a hope, and the brief story of interferon undoubtedly represents the biggest disappointment of the immunologists in recent years.

The phenomenon of virus interference played an important part in the story of the common cold. As a phenomenon it had been known for many years that the presence of one virus already established will prevent or slow down the growth of a second virus in the infected tissue or the infected animal. Indeed, it was known that even the presence of killed or inactivated virus would prevent the success of a second invader. But by an odd coincidence it was almost exactly at the same time that virus interference was helping progress in identifying the cause(s) of the common cold that the true explanation of the phenomenon was discovered. In 1957 Dr. Alick Isaacs, working in London with a Swiss collaborator, Dr. Lindemann, showed that the presence of virus in a cell caused the cell to produce a substance—they named it "interferon"—which prevented the growth of other virus.

The techniques they used take us right back in the history of immunology to the work on growing influenza virus in eggs. Isaacs, a young man at the time of his discovery, treated chick embryos with large doses of inactivated 'flu virus, having used mild heat or ultraviolet light to reduce the infectivity of the virus. After a few hours the new substance, interferon, was released into the fluids of the eggs. When the membranes of fresh eggs were dosed with this substance, they resisted the growth of active, live influenza virus. Here, then, was a mechanism, previously quite unknown, by which cells would fight a virus infection.

Furthermore, here was the explanation of the body's resistance to the first attack of any virus. All immunological clinical practice has been built on the understanding that once we have had one attack of measles we have a strong resistance to any further attack. But on first meeting a new virus antigen it is several days, perhaps a week, before any large amount of circulating antibody can be detected in the blood—that is, quantities of antibody sufficient to control and subdue the disease. (We have also seen that cell-mediated response is aroused much more quickly and is normally dying down in its intensity before the full antibody defence is mounted.) The fact that the body seemed to have no natural, quickly acting defence against virus had long been a puzzle, although it was known that the injection of small doses of infective agents did not necessarily lead to a full-scale attack of the disease. Interferon supplied the answer.

The obvious implication of the discovery of interferon was very exciting. Surely it should be possible to provide extra supplies of interferon to anyone suspected of being infected by virus and thus to overwhelm the virus by the natural defensive substance before it had a chance to gain hold? The therapeutic possibilities seemed enormous.

The early research seemed entirely favourable. In experimental infections with live and active virus, interferon started to appear within a few hours of the infective injection.

The amount of interferon could then be seen to increase roughly parallel with the increase of virus until the growth of virus was stopped and the amounts began to fall. Only then did the amount of interferon being produced also start to fall. By then the first of the large numbers of antibodies had begun to appear. Interferon really was the cell's natural defence mechanism against invasions which actually penetrated the cell wall.

Even better, at least for the hopes of a major new therapy, various different viruses caused cells to produce the same type of interferon; thus interferon was not like antibodies in being specific for each kind of disease. Then, by irradiating animals with X-rays so as to knock out their immune system and prevent the formation of antibodies at least for a time, it was clearly demonstrable that interferon enabled them to recover from a normal infection. Interferon was shown to be the normal first line of defence against virus, and antibody, which is itself the first line of defence against bacteria, simply acts as a preventive measure against further attacks by the same virus—not least because the antibody, once formed, can attack the virus before it gets into cells, while it is still circulating.

But after this wonderfully hopeful start to the story of interferon, the disappointments began. At first it seemed as though there was simply a slowing down in research. Interferon was remarkably difficult to handle; it was difficult to obtain any large quantities of the material; it was even more difficult to get pure interferon. The substance was easy to separate from the virus it was attacking because interferon could resist the effects of acids strong enough to disintegrate the virus. But it was by no means so easy to separate the interferon from other cell products which were inevitably there when a cell attacked by virus, and therefore one which was producing interferon, was broken up in the laboratory for study.

Today, fourteen years after the discovery of interferon, we still do not know exactly what it is. We can only say that it is a protein which appears to have two different forms distinguishable only by their weight. Still less have we any knowledge as to how interferon works, and how it attacks the virus. There is little more than a suggestion that interferon causes some other substance to be produced and that this secondary substance interferes with the ability of the virus to use the ribosomes inside the cell for manufacturing components of further virus particles. (The ribosomes are small pieces of cellular machinery used in the process of actually linking up amino acid building blocks to make proteins, enzymes, and other complicated biochemicals acting on the instructions of the nucleic acid code.)

And when the problem, the purely technical problem, of obtaining highly purified interferon had been provisionally solved, the big disappointment followed. It turned out that

interferon was "species-specific." That is to say, human interferon is only made by human cells and it only works in
human cells. Likewise, mouse interferon only works in
mouse cells. This immediately shattered the hopes of being
able to produce large quantities of interferon in animals or
animal cell cultures for use in therapy.

There was a long pause in the work on interferon—and
the tragic death of Alick Isaacs removed the most obvious
source of inspiration to persevere. The next big steps, and the
source of most of the present hope that interferon will still be
useful one day in therapy, came from America, chiefly from
Maurice Hilleman and his team at the Merck Institute of
Therapeutic Research in Rahway, New Jersey.

The broad idea now is to use an interferon inducer, a substance which must be harmless in itself but which will stimulate cells that are not currently under attack by virus to produce quantities of interferon. This will then be available to
stop any virus which does try to spread from an infected cell.
The idea came from the discovery that the natural inducer of
interferon formation is a particular feature of the virus itself.
The most active factor in persuading a cell to start producing
interferon is "double-stranded RNA"—two intertwined,
enormously long spiral molecules that is the genetic material
of many viruses. The discovery explains the original observation that damaged, inactivated, or non-infective virus can
cause interferon to be produced; and indeed damaged virus
seems to be a better provoker of interferon than whole virus.
Damage to a virus presumably involves damage to its outer
coat of protein, which is believed to be responsible for the
function of penetrating cell walls. But damage to the outer
coat would be expected to reveal the inner genetic nucleic
acid material, which in many types of virus is none other
than double-stranded RNA—a satisfying theoretical full
circle.

But Hilleman took his discovery a stage further. He produced a non-infective copy of double-stranded RNA, a material called Poly I:C. This can best be described as a molecule rather similar to the long molecules that make our modern plastics and man-made fibres, but with a structure like the twin, intertwined strands of RNA. Poly I:C undoubtedly induces cells to manufacture interferon when no virus is present inside them. Indeed, it has been shown to limit the effect of some virus infections in experimental animals. But it obviously cannot in its present form be considered for therapeutic use, because it must be injected and has unacceptable side-effects. This research is at present working on improving the effects of Poly I:C by chemically modifying the molecule.

In the late summer of 1970 an important and stimulating step forward was taken with the discovery of a different interferon inducer. This is a totally separate kind of molecule, a coal-tar derivative called tilorone hydrochloride. Krueger and Mayer of the Merrell Company at Cincinnati, backed by work from Merigan and his team at Stanford University, have shown that this compound, although a small molecule, seems to be highly effective in inducing interferon production. They claim to have shown that it has prophylactic value against nine different viruses in animals, yet it has very little side-effect. It is reported that trials with human subjects are under way.

And in the last few months of 1970 came a flood of new ideas, new discoveries, new techniques, which lead one to hope that interferon may soon be omitted from a discussion about the failures of immunology.

Firstly, one of the technical problems of producing large amounts of interferon for study is that some forms of interferon are highly unstable. Soon after the interferon has been manufactured by a cell, it is chemically broken down into its constituent parts. Although interferon found in animal blood serum is perfectly stable, even if it is hard to purify and only present in small quantities, the interferon produced in the laboratory by tissue cultures of cells, though in large quantities, is unstable and rapidly broken down. No one knows why this difference should occur, but an extremely simple way of dealing with it has been discovered by Graff and Kassell of the Columbia-Presbyterian Medical Center in New York. They simply add blood serum (from horses) to the interferon produced by their laboratory cell-cultures (actually mouse cell-cultures). The result, inexplicably, is stable interferon.

Another major step forward has been the discovery by Professor Ernst Chain's Department of Biochemistry at Imperial College in London, of a naturally occurring virus, which normally attacks fungi, but which can also be persuaded to induce the production of interferon by the penicillium mould organism. There is a fascinating irony here, for Professor Chain's place in the history of science is as one of Florey's team of young biochemists at Oxford University. In the late 1930's and early 1940's, this team succeeded in transforming penicillin from a laboratory curiosity to the world's first antibiotic. And now, thirty-odd years later, Professor Chain has found that the penicillium organism with which he has worked all his life can in fact be infected with a virus, and can be induced to produce yet another valuable therapeutic substance.

A virus that attacks a fungus has now been labelled a "mycophage," to the regret of those of us who liked the euphonious "fungiphage." But the culture and development of this virus, and the attempt to use it to induce the production of commercial quantities of interferon, has now been taken up by the pharmaceutical industry. Since the virus essentially consists of double-stranded RNA, it has an obvious advantage over synthetic chemicals as an inducer of interferon, because the evidence points to RNA as the natural inducer of interferon in normal circumstances. The drug company that has been entrusted by the National Research Development Corporation with the development of Professor Chain's discovery in Britain is the Beecham Research Laboratories. This organisation has discovered the nucleus of penicillin, 6-amino-penicillanic acid, and from this has gone on to world leadership in the development and manufacture of semi-synthetic penicillins—antibiotics "tailored" at the molecular level to perform specific jobs.

Parallel with these developments in the production of quantities of interferon, have come more and more encouraging reports about the therapeutic effects of the substance. From France, Ion Gresser and his colleagues at the Institut de Recherche Scientifique sur le Cancer, have reported a considerable degree of protection from cancer by interferon in mouse experiments. In control mice, untreated with interferon but inoculated with tumour cells, only 7 out of 188 survived for 22 days and none lived for more than 60 days; 103 mice were given similar injections of tumour cells but also received interferon, and 101 survived beyond 22 days and 16 lived beyond the 60-day mark.

Graff and Kassell, mentioned above, have also reported encouraging results against mouse leukaemias and other cancers. Those who are following Hilleman's work at the Merck Institute for Therapeutic Research, along the avenues opened up by the interferon-inducing powers of Poly I:C, are finding distinct anti-tumour effects by simply applying the Poly I:C to cancerous animals and letting the interferon induction go on inside the experimental animals. These encouraging results may be accounted for not only by inducing extra interferon by the Poly I:C, but may be, to some extent, produced by the Poly I:C stimulating the immune system in general, or even having an anti-tumour effect of its own.

In many laboratories, the protective effects of interferon are now being studied in connection with many more diseases than cancer. The results are generally so encouraging that the next few years will surely see interferon finally removed from the category of failures.

Malaria

Malaria is the most important infectious disease in the world today; it is perhaps significant of my own European parochialism that I have left it until last in my list of the failures of immunology.

But in giving precedence to the common cold and to interferon, I suspect I am only reflecting the attitude of the immunologists. For most of the present generation of immunologists malaria presents a problem of which they are unaware or only just becoming aware. Their predecessors looked at malaria very closely in the 1920's and 1930's. Then twenty years ago it seemed as if malaria was beaten. We had effective personal prophylactic drugs, which any Westerner could take when he entered malarial countries, and which many Westerners as soldiers were forced to take when they were sent to the Far East or Africa. The highly effective insecticides, DDT and its chemical relatives, were sweeping away the mosquitoes long known to be the carriers of the disease. Enormous programs of malaria eradication based on the use of insecticides were launched by whole nations, backed by the United Nations and supported by money, experts, and techniques from the developed countries. Many of these programs, for example the one in Ceylon, have been notable successes, and it has been estimated that 1,000 million people have had the curse of malaria lifted from their lives and countrysides as a result. For twenty years, therefore, malaria has been a matter for the public health expert, for the international civil servant, for governments and health services and pharmaceutical industries. Not for the immunologist.

But now the mosquitoes are becoming resistant to the insecticides and the malarial organisms are becoming resistant to the drugs, a fact shown rather alarmingly among U.S. troops in Vietnam. Even more important—because new insecticides and new drugs can be developed if we wish—is the steady diminution of the political wish to pursue nation-wide anti-malaria campaigns among the very poorest countries, where the desire for advance in education, in agricultural production, and in economic strength competes against the proposal that the elimination of a single disease will be more beneficial to the health and welfare of the community. So the question of a vaccine against malaria has suddenly come to the fore again within the past three or four years.

Probably the best index of scientific interest in a subject is the simple one of the number of papers describing its research. A recent review of the subject of anti-malarial vaccines shows that between 1946 and 1966 there was only one important paper in the international scientific journals. But then in 1966, '67, and '68 the papers started to flow again, and once more groups of scientists all round the world were back at work injecting chickens, rabbits, and monkeys with various different extracts of malarial organisms and examining their reactions, very much in the way that Pasteur, his colleagues, and contemporaries had worked.

There is, however, a big difference between malaria and the diseases caused by bacteria and virus. The organism causing malaria is plasmodium. There are many different types of plasmodium; plasmodium falciparum is the commonest cause of human malaria, but there is also plasmodium malariae, plasmodium vivax, and the many animal malarias, such as plasmodium berghei, plasmodium knowlesei, and plasmodium gallinaceum. These plasmodia are not simple bacteria which reproduce themselves by splitting into two. They are larger, more complicated creatures, with a complex life cycle, including sexual and asexual stages. And at one stage of their lives they spread themselves by producing what can best be described as spores.

Their effect inside human beings is also essentially different from the effect of a bacterial invasion. Plasmodia are in fact parasites. They parasitise particularly the red cells of the blood. It is this that gives the symptoms and often the fatalities of the disease humanity has known for thousands of years as malaria. But other phases of the plasmodium life cycle also take place inside the human body, involving liver cells and the spreading of the organism in its early stages of development through the blood stream. The discovery of the full complexity of the life cycle of plasmodium falciparum has been comparatively recent. Until twenty years ago it was not understood that the malarial organism differed greatly in its behaviour from ordinary bacteria; and although it is still true that the carrier of malaria is the mosquito, it is now also known that the malarial organism is carried infectiously from one human being to another by the mosquito only at one stage of its development. Indeed, the plasmodium seems to have adapted its developmental timing so that its infectious stage is more common in the blood stream at those times of the twenty-four-hour day when mosquitoes are most likely to bite men.

As the infective agent has several stages in its development, it follows that different antigens are present at different times. The whole problem of immunity to plasmodia thus immediately becomes complicated. The immunologist is also faced with the theoretical problem, in terms of the science of self, that in those parts of the world, such as West Africa, where malaria is endemic, the people carry malarial parasites in their blood virtually throughout their lives. They also carry antibody to the parasites in pretty large quantities at the same time, so that the usual situation of antibody attacking antigen and eliminating it just does not seem to be happening.

The most likely explanation of this state of affairs—the one which seems most supported by evidence—is that the antibody cannot get at the parasites which are inside the red blood cells, but that there is enough antigen continually around from dying cells and dying parasites to keep the antibody level up high. The antibody then provides a protective immunity, an immunity against "super-infection," holding the parasites at at least a fairly controlled level, ready to deal with any upsurge in the disease, and possibly also exerting an "antitoxic" effect and keeping the symptoms of the disease under control.

Broadly speaking, it seems that a child born in an area where malaria is endemic arrives in the world fairly well protected by antibodies received from its mother. But as this passive immunity wears off, the child is usually attacked by the plasmodia. Up to the age of about three, the parasite appears to have its best chance of killing the child, because after that age the amount of antibody starts increasing steadily, reaching its maximum levels at about twenty to twenty-five. But there are some unusual features even about this fairly average picture. It seems very odd that for the first two years the antibody is largely of the IgM type, whereas later on in the process the IgG antibody appears to play a larger and larger role.

It is quite possible that there are unknown numbers of different strains and varieties even within one species of plasmodium. It has been suggested that continual infection with one species, say plasmodium falciparum, may be achieved by continuous reinfection with different antigenic variants (much as the common cold manages to keep circulating in more northerly climes). Alternatively, the plasmodia may have the ability to vary their antigens in rather the same way that the influenza virus manages to persist by continually re-appearing in fresh antigenic disguises. On the other hand, it is clear that most human antibodies to malaria are antibodies to the "fully grown" parasite, that is, to the stage of development when the plasmodium is a parasite within the red blood cells. It has been shown to be experimentally possible to make antibodies to some of the other stages of the life cycle, but antibody to these stages is not usually found in human beings suffering from malaria. Even further complications enter the picture when some of the antibodies formed during malarial infections appear to be quite "inert"; they cannot be found to be doing anything at all. A suggested explanation for the presence of these inactive antibodies is that in the complex relations between parasites and cells, especially in the disintegration of cells, fresh antigens may be exposed or even entirely new substances with new antigenic properties produced.

Cell-mediated immune reactions may or may not be present in dealing with malarial infections. Professor Ian Mc-Gregor, head of the Medical Research Council's unit in Gambia, West Africa, says simply: "Although considerable progress has been made in the field of humoral immunity, the study of the cellular basis of malarial immunity has languished in the past twenty years." Only in the past twenty years has the modern concept of cell-mediated immunity arisen; and the first papers to link malarial immunity with cellular action started to appear only in 1968. But it has been shown that neo-natal thymectomy increases the susceptibility of rats to malaria. And it has long been known that enlarged spleens are a common symptom in continuous malarial infection, which is significant since the spleen has come to be recognised as one of the important lymphoid tissues.

The presence of large numbers of different antigens in cases of malarial disease has complicated the study of immunity against plasmodia: the preparation of vaccines against malaria becomes an even more difficult problem. But the immunologists have been busy, at least since 1966 and 1967, in trying out various possible immunisation techniques long before they have discovered all about the disease. This is not only in the best traditions of their predecessors but gives yet another illustration of the way in which immunology breaks from the classical myths about scientific procedure.

A great many chickens, mice, rats, and monkeys have been inoculated with all sorts of plasmodial materials and fractions of the serum of other infected animals. Many results showing good degrees of protection against one strain or another of the plasmodia have been reported; in addition, protection has been reported against various different stages in the life cycle of the parasite. What do these results mean in practical terms? Professor McGregor, in his most recent report, says: "It is too early to assess the significance of the many interesting results that are currently emerging from animal experimentation, nor is it clear how much of the new knowledge can be applied to the problem of immunising man against malaria." [2] He then refers to a factor which has cropped up again and again in the story of immunology: the need for a laboratory method of cultivating the plasmodia parasites so that they can be studied properly. In this case we need not only a method of growing the plasmodia in the laboratory but some means for growing them in all the different stages of their life cycles.

So far the results from vaccination experiments appear to favour the likelihood of the eventual answer being a live, attenuated vaccine, in which the plasmodium is still a living organism, but with its infectivity and its capacity to parasitise red blood cells reduced to completely safe levels by continuously passaging it from one animal to another, or from one culture to another, for many generations. An interesting variation on the usual progress towards a vaccine, however, has risen in the case of malaria. It arose from the suspicion that part of man's immune response to malaria is an antitoxic immunity, which means that some of the work of the antibodies is to mop up dangerous substances resulting from the action of the parasites, as well as to attack the parasites themselves. Dr. Jerusalem infected one set of mice with malaria (plasmodium berghei) and on the seventh day of their infection extracted blood from them. With serum from this blood he injected a second, uninfected group. Then he infected the second group of mice with plasmodium berghei. The immunised mice developed much greater numbers of parasites in their blood, carried them for much longer, and survived for greater periods than untreated mice who had been infected at the same time with the same parasite.

The suggestion is that the immunised mice were protected against some unknown toxic product of the parasites. Because of this protection they were able to survive longer than unprotected mice, and this survival in its turn gave the parasites time to increase their numbers to higher levels in the protected mice. But the longer survival with the larger number of parasites also gave the protected mice time to mount much more powerful immune defences and thus they were also able to survive the longer period overall. Such are the complications of anti-malarial immunology studies.

The search for a vaccine and the basic research into malarial immunities are not, however, quite the end of the connection between malaria and immunology. There is a growing suspicion that infection with malaria can lead to other disease states which may well be caused by auto-immune reactions. Once again it is pointed out that there are large numbers of different antigens involved in the plasmodial life cycle and probably further antigenic material produced by the complex reactions of host and parasite. It would not be surprising if some of the antibodies produced against this barrage of antigen also turned out to be harmful to the body.

The suspicion began when blackwater fever, a dreaded complication of malaria prevalent right up to the time of the Second World War, suddenly declined very rapidly after the new synthetic drugs replaced quinine for the treatment of malaria in the 1940's. Add to this the long-known facts about enlarged spleens in cases of malaria and that really badly enlarged spleens (tropical splenomegaly) only seem to occur in malarial areas, and there is foundation for suspicion.

More recently it has been found that there is definite clinical evidence to link a kidney disease (glomerulonephritis) with attacks of malaria caused by plasmodium malariae. There is evidence supporting the idea that antibody/antigen complexes (that is, lumps of antibody bound to antigen) may be deposited in the kidney tissues, where they cause the original damage of glomerulonephritis. This of course links closely with the suspicions about the damaging role of antibody/antigen complexes in other auto-immune diseases such as rheumatoid arthritis. There is also a growing body of opinion that the anaemia associated with malaria infections is more severe than can be accounted for by the destruction of red blood cells by the parasites themselves. There is evidence that parasite antigens can become attached to red cells which are not themselves invaded by the parasites, but which would obviously therefore come under attack by antimalarial antibodies. There is also evidence that auto-antibodies to heart, thyroid, and gastric tissues can be found in some cases of malaria. (I have ignored the equally fascinating but non-immunological subject of the genetics of natural resistance to malaria.)

The simple conclusion must be that the immunology of

malaria is at present just too complicated for us to understand, and too detailed for current methods of identification and measurement to sort out without many years of hard work. In those years a vaccine may well emerge before we have gained a full understanding of the relationships between plasmodia and the human body. But the fact that malaria is the world's most prevalent major infectious disease is a measure of the immunologists' failure to concentrate enough resources in this one field, as well as of their success in dealing with other infectious diseases.

Chapter 11

The Future
of Immunology

It is impossible to predict the future of science. Any good scientist will tell you that. The whole point of science is to find out new things and make discoveries. If scientists could predict what they were going to find in the future there would be no point in going on to do the work. Even more important, there would be no fun, no excitement, in science. I have heard a good many famous scientists speak to this effect. I remember particularly Francis Crick's lecture to celebrate the centenary of *Nature*, during which he elaborated a series of predictions, some obviously very seriously thought out, others highly amusing. Advancing precisely from the premise of the unpredictability of science, he suggested that we must consider the possibility of the development of the most unlikely new disciplines. On this basis, if I remember correctly, we can expect a science of molecular theology to spring up.

But the point about the unpredictability of scientific advance, though valid, is merely a caveat. The scientist always provides his share of predictions. I shall follow in well-known footsteps and give mine.

There are, in fact, a number of sound bases on which one

can usefully make predictions. One can take those areas about which there is most debate at the moment and reasonably suggest that someone will come up with some of the answers in the near future. Or one can take those areas in which there is at present the most progress, the fastest movement, and the greatest excitement, and reasonably predict what the developments are likely to be, because in these areas the most advanced workers do have a glimpse of what they and their colleagues are working towards. Yet another reasonably sound method of prediction is to ask the scientists what field they themselves would like to move into. Since the essence of good science is to have some good questions to ask of nature, it is likely that the questions that are just beginning to formulate in the minds of the scientists are going to provide some interesting answers. Finally, one can adopt the more practical line of questioning used in the budding science of technological forecasting.

Technological Forecasting

Technological forecasting is much more strongly developed in the United States than in other countries, and certainly it has found very little favour in Britain. Among big companies in the American aero-space and electronics fields it has been well funded and much used; the Honeywell Corporation, for instance, has produced a complex technological forecasting system of its own called "Patterns," which has led the firm to make major changes in its proposals for research investment in systems of inertial navigation. It is in the United States, too, that we find the "temples" of technological forecasting at the Rand Institution. And at the Hudson Institute Hermann Kahn is "high priest."

The strict definition of technological forecasting reads as

follows: "Technological Forecasting is the probabilistic assessment, on a relatively high confidence level, of future technology transfer." This comes from Eric Jantsch, the man who virtually introduced technological forecasting to Europe in a book written for the Organisation for Economic Cooperation and Development (OECD) in 1967, entitled *Technological Forecasting in Perspective.* The crucial part of this definition is "technology transfer." This phrase has a fairly strict mathematical meaning, referring to a graphical representation of "technology transfer space"; but here it suffices to say that it not only implies the movement of technology and its development through time but also refers to the number of people affected by a technology at different times. The rest of the definition can be reduced to "expressing it in figures by using mathematical techniques."

Technological forecasting can be carried out in many different ways, but they all fall into one or other of two categories. There is exploratory forecasting, which means extrapolating from the present state of knowledge. And there is "normative" forecasting, which consists of visualising some future state of affairs and deducing the changes in technology that will be involved in getting there. Thus if one looks for one of the growth points of the science of immunology at the moment, one of those subjects surrounded by excitement and the object of current research, it is reasonable to predict that there will be progress at this point. Furthermore, it is fairly clear what the next immediate advances are likely to be, and from this one can predict what likely clinical benefits may arise. This is exploratory forecasting, extrapolating from the present. It is usually very accurate for the immediate future but tends to get less and less accurate the longer the time range, for obvious reasons. Yet it is also quite valid to imagine a world in twenty years time in which the global population is double its present figure. By then there may well have arisen a demand for some form of compulsory birth control which does not violate human rights and dignity as much as compulsory sterilisation, yet is more effective than self-administered pills, or diaphragms, or IUDs. Compulsory immunisation of women against all male sperm or against an individual husband's sperm after the production of the second child might be a possibility for technological development. This is normative forecasting, and it is probably more accurate over a long-term range than exploratory forecasting.

The present aim of the technological forecasters is to find some way of combining the forward projection of exploratory forecasts with the backward projection of normative forecasts, while at the same time allowing for the "crosswind" effects of unknown future discoveries in totally different disciplines. It is also fairly clear that at present exploratory forecasting is based largely on technical and technological possibilities, whilst normative forecasting tends to be more concerned with social or sociological points of view. There is some hope that sociological research into the impact of new technologies now affecting our societies will provide clues as to how we might join up the forward end of the exploratory forecast with the rearmost point of the normative forecast. In any event, a considerable amount of academic research is now going on with the objective of improving the techniques of technological forecasting.

Despite the comparative backwardness of Britain in this business, the most interesting recent application of technological forecasting to the medical field was organised there, although it used the knowledge and intelligence of men from the United States, Sweden, and Holland as well as native experts. This was the forecast called *Medicines in the 1990's* already mentioned in Chapter Two, prepared by the Office of Health Economics. It was produced by the "Delphi" method, which is a very sophisticated and highly controlled form of crystal-gazing. Forty experts were asked for their forecasts on a range of subjects, together with their estimates of the chief obstacles to progress, and their ranking of the problems on a scale of difficulty. The forty sets of answers were then consolidated where possible, and over the other points the conflicting forecasts were set out. Next, this draft was circulated to the experts for their comments. Some of the forecasts were rejected as invalid by specialists in particular fields and each one of the forty was able to help in the clarification and development of the total forecast. A final round of consultation produced the end result.

The final forecast covers a much wider field than the science of immunology. It groups disease states into nineteen main "families" and even looks briefly at the future of veterinary medicine. Nearly half of the forecast deals with the social rather than the clinical aspects of medicine—there are forecasts covering the future of the British National Health Service, the future of the pharmaceutical industry, the future of medical finance, and public and preventive health, and so on. Naturally, too, there are forecasts about the increased use of computers in aiding diagnosis, leading to much wider programs for "screening" the general public. Some of the most interesting aspects of the forecast appear in these sections; for instance, there is the suggestion that by the start of the next century medicines will be available to speed the learning processes, improve dexterity, counter stress or fatigue, and modify our perception of our surroundings. In thirty years time such medicines may well be publicly accepted for social purposes and they are quite likely to be welcomed as safer alternatives than our present social drugs such as alcohol, tobacco, and marijuana.

The final report on the forecasts is quite frank about the fact that the greatest conflict among the individual predictions came in the field of cancer, where opinions were sharply divided between optimists and pessimists. Said the optimists: "Work on the immune aspects of graft rejection and on immune responses to certain cancers may also produce quite rapid results. Indeed both specific and non-specific means of stimulating the body's immune responses (in this context its cancer-rejection mechanisms) are foreseen by 1980." The gloomy view of the pessimists was that "new cancers will emerge, possibly as fast as existing ones are dealt with, and these new cancers will prove extremely difficult to control."

I mentioned the various vaccines against specific infectious diseases when referring to these forecasts in Chapter 2. In more general terms the experts agree that vaccines will come to play a larger and larger part in our lives as the twentieth century progresses and as preventive medicine becomes more and more widespread. Indeed, they foresee our reliance on vaccines becoming even greater than "steady progress" would predict because the amount of "natural immunity" in our populations will decrease as more and more of the common infectious diseases are virtually eliminated; our continued protection against these diseases will then come to depend almost totally on vaccination.

Immunology figured most largely when the forecasters turned their attention to the problems of grafting. They rated the overcoming of graft rejection as "difficult" or "very difficult" and there was even the extreme view that "the body mechanisms involved are so fundamental to human survival that their suppression might even prove impossible." The majority, however, favoured "significant" progress by 1975 and "major" progress by 1980.

Speaking of further problems of immunology the report says:

> An improved anti-lymphocyte serum is thought to be the first likely product of research, but improvements in tissue-

typing and in the banking of organs will not be much slower. A more important advance, however, based upon a much better understanding of the basic phenomena of rejection, will be the production of immuno-suppressive agents of enhanced specificity, which will suppress the undesired immune response while leaving unaffected the general immunological process. Possibly of equal importance will be the development of biological methods of producing immunological tolerance for a specific tissue, again while leaving the general immunological process unaffected.[1]

The experts go on to reject as impossible the idea of breeding an animal whose tissues will be compatible with the great variety of human tissue types. But in the exceptional cases of babies with congenital heart disease they forecast that by 1975 the first attempts may be made to produce artificial tolerance (of the Medawar type) by injecting the baby with animal tissue just before or just after birth and later giving an organ graft from the same type of animal. Two other individual forecasts in this field are interesting: the suggestion that heart transplants will be widely used by as early as 1975 on the one hand; and on the other, the view that an ability to graft teeth and skin with ease will prove of more value in relieving human suffering than heart transplantation.

Another section in which immunological progress figures largely is that on diseases of the connective tissues. In general the outlook in this field is not held to be promising, the reason being the lack of general immunological knowledge:

> There are a great variety of serious basic difficulties: One is the need to understand the basic mechanics of cell membranes and cell enzymes, although these may be controllable by 1985; another is the need for a greater knowledge of the immunochemical reactions involved, and of the immunoglobulin precursors (that is of those substances that will form

antibody in response to the presence in a person's body of an antigen).[2]

Yet a third basic difficulty enunciated by the forecasters, though not strictly immunological, emphasises a problem to which I have referred several times here: the problem of reproducing rheumatoid arthritis in animals by any process which could conceivably operate in man. They conclude: "Nevertheless by 1980 we may at least have clarified the role of infection in initiating and of an immune process in perpetuating rheumatoid arthritis. . . . The main therapeutic problem is to develop medicines that will interfere selectively with antigen-antibody formation."

In contrast to the gloomy outlook on connective tissue diseases, the forecasters expect steady progress against only "moderate difficulties when it comes to dealing with allergic disorders." Fundamental advances, they agree, will only come from immunological research, and they particularly mention the importance of characterising the immunoglobulin of allergy, IgE. They expect that this fundamental research will take up to 1980 but that in the 1980's there will begin to be major therapeutic fruits. They append, however, a warning that technological advances in other fields, bringing us new foods and new general utilities as well as new medicines, will at the same time bring new allergens into our lives and they expect that we shall always retain the basic liability to suffer from allergic reactions.

Two final points about this fascinating glimpse into our medical future. The experts expect immunisation against pregnancy to be available by 1975 (and here I feel they are very optimistic) and they make no mention of possible immunological impact on the research into the process of ageing.

Whether or not one believes that technological forecasting will turn out to be a useful guide to investment and management in research, its techniques are certainly the soundest basis we have at the moment for looking into the future. I shall therefore take the main items of immunological interest from *Medicines in the 1990's* as the guide for my own predictions in the remainder of this chapter, and I shall endeavour to show in rather greater detail the sort of work and thinking that lies behind some of these predictions. But whereas the technological forecasters approached their problems within the framework of a general concept of medicine as a social phenomenon, I shall take as my starting points those matters that are arousing the greatest interest and excitement among immunologists and do my quota of "exploratory forecasting" by extrapolating from these points.

Probably the most puzzling single feature of the theories of the science of self is the problem of accounting for the enormous variety of antibodies which the body is prepared to make right from the start of the working of the immune system. The theory, of course, is that there are at least some small lymphocytes carrying antibody against every possible antigen that can ever be met. These lymphocytes, with their specific antibody to every possible antigen, must be produced by the body before it has met and recognised any of the antigens. This demand of the theory is not quite so enormous as it may seem at first sight, because antigens and antibodies are primarily "shapes" at the molecular level and there is some pattern, some relatedness, between the various kinds of molecule that go to make up living things, at least on this planet in the type of life forms we know.

But there are two rival theories concerning the development, within every growing body, of the huge variety of antibodies necessary if that body is to face all the many assaults that may be made on its selfhood and integrity. One school of thought—the original Burnet line—holds that at some stage of development there is a sudden tremendous outburst of variation in the bone marrow cells, the stem cells that will later produce the lymphocytes. This somatic variation (in this case, "somatic" meaning at the level of the whole cell) implies that there must be some force or factor at this stage of development which can cause a cell capable of making one type of antibody to produce daughter cells which are capable of making different types of antibody. And so on, until there are cells present which can make every type of antibody. This is where the little joke about GOD— the generator of diversity—comes in.

The rival theory holds that the production of all these different sorts of antibody is controlled, like all other cellular manifestations, by the nucleic acids. This in turn implies that the huge amount of information needed to code for the production of all the antibodies is carried in the long spirals of DNA which make up our chromosomes. The question arises whether there is room on the chromosomes for all the information required. At first sight this seemed hardly possible. But with the knowledge that such large portions of the immunoglobulins, in the shape of heavy chains and light chains, were similar, and that the variations in antibody were largely confined to the actual binding sites at the end of the chains, the sheerly mathematical difficulties of packing all the information onto just so much DNA were reduced. Furthermore, it began to be possible to visualise evolutionary schemes in which first heavy chains were evolved with variations only at the binding site, and then light chains were evolved, and so on, with just one stretch of DNA coding providing most of the information required for these chains.

Recently, while the earlier chapters of this book were being written, several papers and publications outlining possible explanations for the production of all the antibodies under the control of nucleic acid have appeared. None of them can be regarded as conclusive. In the words of one of the best-known theorists in this field, "Shares in somatic variation have been slumping and shares in genetic control have been improving, but neither set of shares dominates the market and there's been no takeover." [3]

Recent work by Cesar Milstein at the Medical Research Council's Molecular Biology Laboratories at Cambridge (England), which I was able to see in the spring of 1971, seems to be rapidly elucidating this problem, and to be providing a compromise answer half-way between the "diversification" and "genetic" theories.

So here is an area in which one can reasonably safely predict that there will be progress in the coming years. This is not to say that one theory or the other will definitely sweep the field. It is quite possible there may be a compromise solution. It may be, for instance, that as we come to understand more about the actual shapes and structures of antigen and antibody, the problem of variation could be reduced in complexity; and it could turn out that a basic set of antibody shapes is provided under genetic control. The final perfect fit against an invader may be provided by rapid selection processes (using "selection" in an evolutionary sense) among the proliferating lymphocytes which have started by carrying an antibody that is at least a good enough fit to the antigen to cause triggering off.

The safest of all predictions in the field of immunology is that great progress will be made in the near future in the study of the detailed structure and activity of immunoglobulins, the antibodies themselves. The two key names in this field are Gerald Edelman, of Rockefeller University in the United States, and R. R. Porter, of the University of Oxford in England—again preserving a nice transatlantic balance.

Other key figures, however, are nameless; they are the individuals unfortunate enough to suffer from myeloma. Their contribution to science and human welfare lies in their having developed what is essentially cancer of the plasma cells, where one plasma cell suddenly starts proliferating madly and pouring enormous quantities of the single antibody it manufactures into the body. Only by recovering this antibody from the serum and urine of these patients can the immunologists obtain sufficient quantities of any one type of immunoglobulin to analyse the molecule chemically.

Porter, as we have seen in an earlier chapter, essentially established the structure of immunoglobulin. Edelman played a major role in those early stages only seven to ten years ago, but his greatest achievement came just in 1969, when he provided the first ever analysis of an immunoglobulin in terms of its constituent amino acids.[4]

The analysis of a single immunoglobulin was a colossal task. It was the largest protein to be so analysed, containing 19,996 atoms making up a sequence of 214 amino acids. The analysis confirmed the general structure of the immunoglobulins, showing variable ends to both the light and heavy chains at one end of the molecule (the binding sites) and long sequences of constant regions at the other end. One by-product of this work is the growth of interest in accounting for the whole production of all the variety of antibodies under the control of the genetic material in the nucleic acid and the construction of evolutionary "schemes" which will account for the development of long constant chains with fine variations at the ends.

But looking at antibodies on the larger scale of examining the entire molecule, as in Porter's work, is producing a welter of "classes," "types," and "subtypes," according to the variations which turn up in the constant portions of the light and heavy chains. In other words, it is possible to identify a number of antibodies which are of the IgG type but of the class, say, "K,1." In this class and type the heavy and the light chains are identical in all members at their constant ends, although they will vary at the binding sites to be specific for different antigens. Different immunoglobulins may be IgG "K,2," in which all the heavy and light chains are again the same within the class and type at their constant ends, but differ in various ways from the constant ends of IgG "K,1."

Presumably these many varieties of immunoglobulins have differing functions. The sorting out of this complicated picture is undoubtedly one of the chief tasks of the chemists and immunologists in the years ahead. Probably a bonus lies at the end of it, in that defining the function and nature of the different immunoglobulins will almost inevitably illuminate the detailed workings of the system.

At this same level of the submicroscopic some other exciting results concerning antibodies have recently turned up. These come largely from the steadily improving techniques of the electron microscopists. As they achieve greater and greater resolution in their pictures, they can now show that an immunoglobulin molecule adopts a slightly different shape when it binds to antigen: when binding takes place the two long arms of the molecule swing out, so that the angle between them becomes greater. It also appears that the antibody molecule has slightly smaller dimensions when it is bound than when it is free. No one really knows yet what this change of shape is, or what it means. But some extremely exciting possibilities are opening up.

One point that has definitely emerged is that this change of shape enables complement to bind to antibody. The combination of complement with antibody is the vital mechanism in the destruction of some cellular invaders by the immune system—that is to say, it is a mechanism chiefly used in defeating bacteria rather than virus invaders. It is not clear precisely what happens, but we know that complement in the presence of antibody literally pierces a hole in the cell wall of the invader. Somehow the change of shape of the immunoglobulin molecule as it binds to the antigen exposes the portion of the immunoglobulin to which complement can bind and achieves this important combination. It is even suggested that the swinging apart of the long arms of the immunoglobulin causes "wrinkles" or "rucks" in the structure of the molecule and that the complement may be able to stick itself onto these wrinkles. It also appears likely that it is on the same part of the immunoglobulin molecule that is used for complement-fixing that antibodies to the immunoglobulin itself can bind.

Here, too, we may possibly have an explanation of "triggering off." There is certainly no clear evidence for this yet, but Edelman has been prepared to speculate[5] that the change in shape of the antibody molecule as it binds to antigen could be the signal to a lymphocyte carrying the antibody to go into the reaction of dividing and multiplying.

Almost every immunologist seems to agree that further detailed study of antibodies is not only essential for progress in most directions in immunology but is also likely to produce valuable new insights into the science of self in the near future. In addition, this field is often mentioned by immunologists as one into which they are considering moving because it offers an exciting junction or interface between chemistry and immunology.

Another favourite subject among practising immunologists as being a likely field for progress is the study of the cytotoxic lymphocyte, the lymphocyte which actually attacks cells on its own account without going into the antibody-manufacturing role. This is a very new branch of the science and there is little that can be said about it at present except that it may provide a valuable lead into the almost unexplored details of the cell-mediated reaction and therefore into the actual mechanism of graft rejection.

Immunology and Ageing

There is no doubt that the phenomenon of ageing is now coming to interest many scientists in many other disciplines as well as immunology. The medical speciality of gerontology is rapidly coming to the fore, if only because there are so many more aged people as the expectation of life increases in our affluent Western communities. But scientists are also wondering why, for instance, salmon age so suddenly after spawning, and it is in the areas of immunology and ageing that Sir Macfarlane Burnet is now putting forward theories. On the general grounds of "form" it is almost certainly worth backing anything in which Burnet is showing an interest.

The immunological theory of ageing, as expounded by R. L. Walford in a book published in 1969,[6] and as subsequently elaborated by Burnet, considers that the basic phenomenon arises in some way from the chance mutation of the ordinary cells of the body. This may be because, with age, the cells more and more often fail to reproduce themselves properly; they copy the genetic instructions with more and more errors as the cell line grows weary. There is also a steadily increasing exposure to the forces of the environment that induce changes in cells.

Normally the mechanism of immunological surveillance should eliminate cells which have either mutated under outside influences or changed through failure to copy the genetic instructions properly. We have considered this mechanism only in connection with the genesis of cancers, but of course there can be non-cancerous mutations of cells. And the changed cells should have different antigens, just as cancerous cells have the different surface antigens identified as tumour specific antigens (TSA). In the case of non-cancerous changed cells, the new antigens may cause auto-immune reactions to start up. The antibody/antigen complexes then formed might have damaging effects on all sorts of tissues (just as they do on the tissues of the joints in rheumatoid arthritis). These damaging effects would increase the speed of ageing even if they were not responsible for the phenomenon directly. At the same time, we can reasonably expect errors to creep into the reproduction of the cells responsible for the immune processes. With changed lymphocytes beginning to roam around, it is then reasonable to expect that some of these would start attacking self tissues, thus giving auto-immune effects and subsequent damage; simultaneously the mechanism of immunological surveillance would be weakened by the random age changes in the lymphoid cells, so that the chances of restricting the damaging effects would also decrease.

The steady increase in the incidence of cancer with age in man, horse, and mouse alike is the strongest evidence that some processes of this type are really happening as an animal grows older. The evidence for the auto-immune effects is not so strong. There is a complicating factor known as the Hayflick effect (after the famous American scientist Hayflick, mentioned before in connection with the development of the technique of tissue culture). One of Hayflick's most surprising and disturbing findings was that a culture of human cells in the laboratory would die for no apparent reason after perhaps as few as twenty generations of cells. Only cancerous human cells will continue to multiply indefinitely in the laboratory. (This must now be qualified somewhat, since Hayflick has managed to get certain rather special lines of human cells to survive more or less indefinitely in culture; these are diploid cells, which have double the normal complement of chromosomes.) No one knows whether the natural death of a line of cells in laboratory glassware also means that cells in a living body will die after one parent cell has produced twenty or so generations of offspring. But it is a good guess that this death of a cell line, the Hayflick effect, probably does occur in the living body too, though the number of generations of cells may be greater in the living system. The best evidence for the existence of the Hayflick effect in the living system is the curious fact that all animals do seem to have a natural life span. This differs from species to species, with smaller animals generally having a shorter span than large animals. Of course some individual animals live longer than other individuals of the same species—we observe this among human beings particularly—but the signs of old age seem to start arriving at about the same time after birth whatever the final age at death of the individual.

Sir Macfarlane Burnet has very recently elaborated, or modified, the basic immunological theory of ageing, by drawing in these extra pieces of evidence and by pointing out the possible significance of the strange fact that, roughly speaking, the thymus, the organ which is so vital to our immune systems, gets smaller throughout life. It is large enough in the young calf to provide us with that notable delicacy, sweetbreads; yet it has almost disappeared by the time old age effects the animal.

The removal of the thymus by surgery does not completely eliminate that half of the immune system which we call thymus-dependent. Nevertheless, it can be reasonably assumed that normally the thymus, even in adult life when it has shrunk so much, is the chief source of new thymus-dependent cells. Yet only 1 percent of all the cells produced in the thymus are eventually released into the rest of the body. In an earlier chapter we noticed this unresolved puzzle about the thymus: that it is packed full of lymphocytes which generate further lymphocytes, but that only a few of the enormous total of thousands of millions of cells are released into the circulation. The point here is not, however, the unexplained oddity of this behaviour; it is that the cell turnover in the thymus—the rate of death and generation of cells—is higher than in any other organ of the body. And this despite the fact that the life of lymphocytes, once they are released from the thymus, may be very long, as long as ten to twenty years. Therefore if there is a Hayflick effect in the living body, the thymus should be the first organ to feel it. The cell lines with which we are born will begin to die off in the thymus before they do so anywhere else.

Immunological surveillance is probably the most important function of the thymus-dependent part of the immune system, and yet if the Hayflick effect really does occur in living systems the thymus should be the first organ to feel the effects of age. It is here that Burnet finds the central cause of the symptoms of ageing. And he summons several impressive lines of evidence to support his theory. Patients with advanced cancer, for instance, show a weakness and inadequacy of the thymus-dependent immune system far more severe than can be accounted for by the simple weakness of ageing. It is just as likely that they have cancer because of a premature weakening of the immune system as that the immune system is weak because they have cancer. And tests on people over sixty-five show that although they can still produce antibody at the normal rate to meet the challenge of any antigen they are known to have encountered in their younger days, they are very slow at, or even incapable of, producing antibody against some specially exotic or unusual antigen. Now this not only accounts for the well-known fact that older people are more susceptible to new infections but may also show that the thymus-dependent system, which is responsible for recognising newly met antigens as not-self, is weakening as the years go on. Similarly, the patterns of auto-immune disease—and particularly the findings of the increasing presence of "anti-self" factors as age increases, even when there is no patent auto-immune disease—strengthen the case.

What practical results will emerge from the development of the immunological theory of ageing is more difficult to assess. Sir Macfarlane Burnet, who is quite old enough to be personally involved in the situation, is gloomy; as he wrote in *The Lancet* in August 1970: "Whether the approach offers any guidance towards the maintenance of a healthy old age in man is more doubtful, but at least it offers a certain rationale for the maintenance of health and the avoidance of 'thymus damaging' stress through the whole of life as the best recipe for a tolerable old age."

Enhancement and Tolerance

The concept of "enhancement" arose from the work on the immunological aspects of cancer. Research experiments aimed at finding out whether cell-mediated immunity or a humoral-antibody immune reaction was most effective against tumours not only revealed that cell-mediated immunity was the chief defence mechanism against cancer cells but also showed that antibody against the tumour cells could actually protect the tumours from attack by the cell-mediated mechanism. Those immunologists interested in clinical work and transplantation surgery seized on the newly discovered phenomenon, and it has recently been applied for the first time in a human case. The patient was a young child (at Guy's Hospital in London) who had suffered from kidney failure at an early age. Because immuno suppression also stunts growth, the primary effect of immuno-suppressive drugs being to stop cell multiplication, there is a special need for techniques that will enable children to receive grafts without the use of the normal drug regime. Some immunologists, in private, criticise the techniques in this first attempt to use enhancement beneficially, and they query the successfulness of the procedures. But they admit nonetheless that the attempt was fully justified and the techniques may yet prove satisfactory in the long run.

While moving into the sphere of practical application, enhancement has also assumed a role of great theoretical interest. It is now believed to be a phenomenon of basic importance in all sorts of immunological reactions. It is the biological technique of immuno suppression regarded as so important by the technological forecast quoted at the start of this chapter. And, as is the way in science, the new concept is being called in as a possible explanation for many puzzling observations. It will probably fail to satisfy all the roles now being thrust upon it, but to some of the puzzles it will surely prove to be the key. Enhancement is bound to become a dominant aspect of that part of the immunological scene that involves transplants and tolerance in the next few years, and there seems no reason to doubt that its further study and use will provide some valuable steps forward.

Probably the most important recent experimental results in the whole field of immunology concern enhancement. The experiments were performed by two Scandinavians, Drs. Karl and Ingegard Hellstrom, now working at the University of Washington in Seattle with a British colleague, Dr. Anthony Allison, another of the foundation staff of the new National Clinical Research Centre in London. In principle, what they have done is to demonstrate particularly clearly the phenomenon of enhancement. They took lymphocytes from patients with a specific type of cancer (neuroblastoma) and mixed them with cells from the same tumour in test tubes. The lymphocytes killed the tumour cells, showing that the patients had in fact been sensitised or immunised by the tumour antigens. But when serum from the same patients was added to the mixture of lymphocytes and tumour cells, the tumour cells were no longer killed. Obviously the explanation is that the serum contains antibody against the tumour cells and this antibody "enhances" the resistance of the tumour cells, probably coating them in such a way that the lymphocytes either cannot recognise or cannot get to the antigenic sites and therefore cannot carry out the cell-mediated immune reaction. Control experiments with lymphocytes and serum from patients without neuroblastoma proved negative.

But then the Hellstroms and Allison carried out similar experiments with mice of two different strains that had been made tolerant to each other by the traditional method. And the surprise came when lymphocytes from an A-strain mouse that had been rendered tolerant to cells from CBA mice successfully attacked tumour cells from a CBA mouse. Further, it was shown that serum from the "tolerant" animal would protect the tumour cells. Finally, they were able to demonstrate that the same results could be obtained the other way round, with CBA lymphocytes, supposedly rendered tolerant to A-strain cells, attacking tumour cells grown in the A strain.

The immediate reaction to these results was a feeling (and some newspaper headlines to the effect) that the traditional theory of tolerance had been severely challenged. But that first surprise has now died down. It is generally felt that there is still ample evidence for the existence of the traditional tolerance, involving the total or virtually total elimination of those clones of cells specific against the antigens of the substance or individual to which the host has been rendered tolerant. But certainly a number of phenomena which have been attributed to the induction of tolerance must in fact be caused by enhancement. Perhaps there is a spectrum of effects. On a mathematical basis, say some 80 percent of the population of lymphocytes specific against some antigen are destroyed. The remainder may either produce such a small reaction quantitatively that enhancement ensues, or may be affected in such a way as to produce slightly altered or deficient antibody which achieves the effect of enhancement without causing the damage of a normal immune reaction.

As soon as the immunologists started reasoning in this way—that there might be a spectrum of resultant effects, varying from complete tolerance through different degrees of protection by enhancement to the full rejection of foreign substances—they thought of various phenomena that might be explained by invoking the action of one part of this spectrum and not the rest. The "decision" as to which portion of the spectrum of reaction might be expected could then very well rest with the actual amount of the provoking antigen that arrived.

For instance there is currently speculation, and it is only speculation, that the phenomenon of successful pregnancy might be explained by enhancement. The steady growth of the amount of foetal antigen—containing the foreign, not-self determinants due to the father's genes, but starting from virtually nothing—might allow the development of maternal antibody sufficient to protect the foetus by enhancement but rarely great enough to cause rejection and consequent abortion. If this line of enquiry proves first viable and then profitable, it could open up an enormous field. For one thing, it might account for the thalidomide tragedy, for it has been suspected that the action of thalidomide was not so much to deform the children of the mothers who took the drug as to prevent the natural abortion of a foetus which would otherwise have been rejected. There are also reasons for thinking that thalidomide, from its chemical nature, might have an immunological action.

Enhancement is also being provisionally called in to provide an explanation for one of the most inexplicable observations to arise out of the progress in transplantation surgery. The observation comes from Professor Roy Calne and his team at Cambridge in England, one of the world's most distinguished and successful liver transplant teams. Though they have now extended their work to providing their first few human patients with transplanted livers, they have done most of their experiments and training on pigs. And the plain fact of the matter is that pigs will accept liver transplants from other pigs and retain the donor liver, working satisfactorily, without any immuno-suppressive drugs and without any apparent attempt to reject the graft. This does not happen every time, but certainly often enough to be a genuine phenomenon, which has to be accounted for and may possibly lead to the discovery of some important new principle or factor at work.

Various attempts have been made to explain away Professor Calne's pig liver results. It has been suggested, for instance, that pigs, being long domesticated and specially bred farm animals, have become so inbred that some of them may be like the genetically pure strains of inbred laboratory mice. But at the London Hospital H. Festenstein of the Transplantation Immunology Unit reported as recently as November 1970 that this is not so and that some real immunological process must be involved. By mixing cultures of lymphocytes taken from the blood of the pigs both before and after the transplantation operation, Festenstein has shown that there definitely is no natural tolerance of donor to host even in cases where the liver transplant has been well received and retained.

The most favoured explanation for this extraordinary state of affairs is that enhancement is somehow induced to protect the graft. But this still leaves open the question of how such rapid enhancement can occur. The explanation, when it is found, may well be exciting and useful. Perhaps Professor Calne will discover some factor peculiar to the liver or manufactured by it which can be induced to come into action strongly and provide enhancement for human liver transplants. But there is still the possibility that the effect may be peculiar to the pig. However, Professor Calne's evidence seems strongly to favour the possibility that the effect has something to do with the liver rather than the pig. For he has transplanted skin, heart, and kidneys from the donor of the liver into the same host, and he has secured, by this means, prolonged retention of the kidney, medium retention of the heart, and least retention of skin. Even so, the skin grafts under these conditions lasted two or three times as long as more normal skin grafts before being rejected. Somehow, it seems, the liver carries its own protective mechanism over to other organs. Grafts of kidneys and skin from other donors were not protected by the grafted liver, except in a few cases.

Enhancement at present is the only process which seems to come anywhere near explaining Professor Calne's results. Even at that it is a little like invoking a magic word to reveal something still unrevealable. But if the liver graft somehow induces enhancement and protection, the mechanism by which it does so could well be usefully applied over a wide number of other cases.

Cancer, Contraception, and Grafting

So far, I have been predicting the future developments of immunology by simple extrapolation of the present trends from the obvious growing points of the science of self. I have picked on those points where there is rapid progress going on at the moment, where new ideas and concepts are beginning to emerge, or which are so exciting that the immunologists themselves are asking new questions. But all across the field of cancer research and treatment there is in fact steady progress. Only a few laymen—and most of us as individuals are frightened of cancer—realise that there has been so much progress in the methods of treatment of many different forms of cancer by the simple improvements in traditional techniques, irradiation and drugs. In addition, there is the continual hope that new and more effective anti-tumour chemicals may be found by chemical research and by the steady screening of new chemicals as they are developed for a wide variety of purposes. A rather more sophisticated approach, currently looking hopeful, comes from the study of the metabolism of cancer cells and the use of chemicals which deprive the tumour cells of some of their special requirements.

This sort of approach, which has nothing to do with immunology, may lead to such successful treatment of most types of tumour that the incentive to pursue the immunological approach dies away. Since cancer is so much more easy to treat and check if it is discovered in the early stages, public health campaigns, screening large numbers of people for the first symptoms of the most common cancers, could actually affect the progress of immunological research. Similarly, the extent to which cancer dominates medical research and individual thinking about health matters could be changed by success in the field of public education, thus reducing the amount of cigarette smoking or other environmental causes of cancer.

But the attempt to implicate viruses as the cause of many cancers is generally regarded among all scientists as one of the most immediately promising lines of cancer research. Viruses have definitely been established as the cause of several bird and animal cancers; it is probably true to say that we are expecting the publication of final, definitive proof that a virus has been incriminated in causing a human cancer literally any day now.

The moment it has been proved that a virus has caused a human cancer, immunology will enter the field. As soon as a virus is identified and isolated, vaccines can, in theory, be prepared against it. Here, a word of warning must be inserted. The ability to prepare a vaccine against a certain virus does not necessarily imply that it will be socially acceptable to vaccinate everyone with it. If the first virus causing human cancers turns up in some rather rare type of cancer, or cannot be found in more than a few patients, it may simply not be economically possible or justifiable to vaccinate millions of people, hundreds of millions of people, on the offchance of protecting a very few against a possible attack by the virus.

In this on the whole rather likely circumstance, a more subtle immunological program may be called for. It is believed that a cancer-causing virus achieves the transformation of a cell into a malignant form by incorporating part of the viral nucleic acid into the genetic material of the cell. This change in the genetic material should be demonstrated externally by a change in antigen on the cell surface which in some way represents the presence of the viral nucleic acid within. A detailed study of these virally transformed cancer cells should lead to the practicability of producing strongly acting antisera or highly responsive cell-mediated reactions against the transformed cells. Some procedure of this sort, or some development of Mathé's immunological treatment of leukaemia, is likely to be the first truly immunological attack upon cancer that we shall see.

There are, however, two other runners in the immunological race against cancer on a broad front (unless you hold that Mathé has already won this race). There is interferon treatment, mentioned in the previous chapter. And there is the possibility of following up the lead that enhancement protects cancerous cells from cell-mediated rejection of a tumour. It ought to be possible to neutralize enhancing anti-

body and thus to expose tumour cells to attack by lymphocytes, although no one has announced any major attempt to
do this experimentally.

Finally, cancers may have to be dealt with by some process involving the action of the immune system as a whole. It
is possible to foresee two ways, in principle, of doing this.
The first is by tightening up the security provided by the
immunological surveillance system; the second, by increasing the avidity of the immune reactions for the weak antigens on the surface of tumour cells, using some variation of
the "helper" theme outlined in Chapter 7.

Contraception by immune methods is undoubtedly a long
way ahead, if it ever arrives at all. And there is not, frankly, a
great deal of practical interest among the leading immunologists in the immune aspects of pregnancy. But the first mur-
murs of speculative interest can be heard now and again.
They come largely from those who feel that the unravelling
of the immunological mysteries involved in pregnancy might
throw light on some of the closer-at-hand puzzles of today's
knowledge of the science of self. But one can be quite sure
that the start of major research efforts into the immunological questions raised by pregnancy will bring to light discoveries of practical importance in dealing with the clinical
problems of reproduction. And that sort of discovery invariably leads to human and widespread social effects.

But in all Western societies, and, one hopes, in developing societies as well, the problem of the aged increases as
medical progress increases the number of individuals who
live up to the full lifespan offered by our genetic equipment.
It would be ridiculous to pretend that immunology can be
anything more than one contributory factor among many in
an approach to providing more and more people with a

happy old age. There is no suggestion that immunological progress can increase the span of life. But there is a possibility that, if the new concepts of there being an immunological factor in the widely known processes of ageing prove to be even partly correct, we could improve the health of the aged. This in turn would much ameliorate the social problems of dealing with the aged. It would provide a work-force for the community with a longer span of active, productive life, and it would decrease the weight on the social services provided by the community by decreasing the number of bed-ridden or housebound. And if wisdom really increases with years, this might be the greatest benefit that immunology will ever bring the human race.

And so to transplants. I am enough of a journalist still to be excited by the dramatic side of transplantation surgery. I am aware that those who work as researchers, immunologists, and surgeons in the field all hope that the great public interest in transplants will die down. I think they are doomed to disappointment. They are like the cavalry of ancient armies, compelled by the very nature of their activity to be spectacular. But I will try to add as little as possible to their burden now by being sober and cautious.

Even so, I can see no very good reason for rejecting the predictions of the best transplant surgeons themselves. Before the end of this century they say that they will be able to transplant kidneys, hearts, livers, lungs, intestines, bone marrow, nerves, skin, and cartilage, and a wide variety of glands or glandular tissues, such as pancreas, thymus, and lymph nodes. And most of the problems of rejection will have been overcome.

There are several routes by which these problems of rejection can be overcome and it seems clear that several of them will prove successful. The immunologists will, for instance, be able to induce tolerance artificially, and there are a number of research programs in many parts of the world that seem reasonably far along the road towards doing this. Then there are the techniques of enhancement to protect the graft and the possibility that someone will find a satisfactory development of antilymphocytic serum (ALS) or some variation on this theme which will lower the immune resistance to the transplant without lowering the status of the whole immune system.

But the likeliest route of all lies in tissue typing. There was considerable disturbance when Paul Terasaki, the outstanding American exponent of tissue typing, produced what seemed to be an extremely gloomy set of figures at the 1970 Hague Transplant Conference. But now that the first shock is over, his colleagues feel that the weakness of his figures was that they contained comparatively few cases from 1970, the vast bulk of the material being provided by pre-1970 cases. Only in the second half of 1970, they feel, has the human tissue-typing problem come anywhere near solution. They are now reasonably confident that there are only four major antigenic determinants at the HL-A locus; and it is these four determinants which between them account for the greater part of human histocompatibility. Extremely good results are being reported for human kidney grafts when these four determinants are well matched between donor and recipient, and highly satisfactory results come from a good match for three of them. There are still puzzles to be sorted out, notably the success of some kidney transplants in cases where donor and recipient appear to be thoroughly bad matches. But there is considerable optimism among the practitioners in the field of tissue typing.

If tissue typing is to be used to its full advantage, however, there must be an increase in the use of computer-controlled matching systems covering fairly large areas of the globe. In practice, at the moment, the areas in which matching schemes of cooperation between numbers of hospitals operate are fairly limited. Although there is officially a Eurotransplant scheme in operation, for instance, it tends to split into two areas, a northwest Europe area, covering Britain, Belgium, and Holland, with Scandinavia on the periphery; and a more southerly area, involving principally northern Italy and France. Considerable improvements in organ storage techniques are desirable if these areas are to be increased in size, so offering better chances of finding good matches between potential recipients and actual donors. But there is no doubt that better organ storage techniques are just round the corner—again there are a number of highly promising research programs afoot. Whether these techniques will be good enough to allow the setting up of organ banks is more problematical, although a number of people involved in this type of research assure me that organ banks will definitely be feasible within five years.

One extremely interesting possible outcome of the work on organ storage is at the moment no more than a glimpse of the future. All organ storage depends on washing out the donor organ as soon as it is removed from the body. This is technically known as perfusion, and the question of the liquid to be used for perfusion and the temperature at which it should be performed are matters of acute controversy among those deeply involved in the work. But there are hints that the most thorough methods, those that remove the maximum amount of donor blood and fluids from the organ, also provide the most satisfactory organs for transplantation. It looks suspiciously as though the more the surgeons can remove of the mobile and easily released donor cells from the organ, the less the rejection reaction.

The long-term future of transplantation surgery lies more in the hands of the multitude of individuals who make up our societies than it does with the surgeon or immunologist.

If transplantation is to become a major feature of our culture, there will have to be a much larger supply of donor organs than there is at present. This is probably not so much a question of religion and ethics as of how individuals really view themselves. The major religious systems of belief and the non-religious systems of ethics seem to offer no objections to transplantation as long as the rights of the donor, perhaps in the last hours of life, are maintained. There are practical problems here but they should not be insuperable. Yet there is undoubtedly a huge inertial load of reluctance to give away our organs or the organs of our relatives when they die. Unless this reluctance can be overcome, interlaced, as it often is, with grief and emotion at the recent death of someone we love and value, transplantation will not become a widespread clinical practice.

In terms of day-to-day politics the argument is whether we should start an "opting-in" scheme or an "opting-out" one. Should we have to declare positively as individuals that we are willing to give our organs when we die? Or should the situation be that surgeons have some actual rights to take over our organs (with safeguards, of course) unless we have positively stated that we do not want to have them removed? Some transplant specialists are campaigning for the second "opting-out" system, but most feel that public opinion, at present at least, will only stand for "opting-in." Any person's attitude to this problem must depend on his attitude towards himself and his body—what he feels about his own integrity of structure. Ironically, it is as if most of us have a mental immune system, a built-in urge to maintain the wholeness of our selves, an irrational need to preserve the integrity of the structure built up on the instructions of our own spiral molecules, even if this means denying a fellow being the chance of life when those spiral molecules can no longer hold together the mass of chemical constituents they have collected from the environment.

Perhaps we do have a mental immune system which also provides the tremendous urge towards self-preservation hitherto regarded as one of the basic psychological factors in the individual. But the immunologists and their science have little to say about it; they are just angry that men will not donate organs to provide the essential material for the life-saving techniques they are making possible. The science of self studies the mechanisms by which an individual system tries to keep its integrity. Only when we philosophise in a thoroughly unscientific manner can we look upon these mechanisms as a definition of the humane self. But the mechanisms can work to the disadvantage of the individual when they break down or are deceived, or when they cannot appreciate the "greater good" that human consciousness can perceive. The science of self, by revealing how these mechanisms work within us, can speed and strengthen their operation as in vaccination to defeat infectious diseases, can correct their failings (at least sometimes), and can override them when the greater good of the individual demands it. But in any science we have to recreate a part of the universe in our own minds in order to discover how it works. And this recreation of our own system of self-preservation is one of the most exciting and fascinating human adventures now in progress.

NOTES

1 Defining the Science of Self

1. (Second ed., London, 1966), p. 304.

2 The Importance of Knowing Who You Are

1. "Disorders of the Immune System," *Hospital Practice*, no. 2 (1967): pp. 38–53.
2. "Symposium on *Lower Animal Neoplasm* 1969," *National Cancer Institute Monograph*, no. 31 (1969): pp. 41–58.
3. See note 1 above.

3 The Mechanism of the Immune System

1. Serum is the liquid, pale yellow and translucent, which is left when the red cells and plasma are extracted from blood. The serum contains the antibodies which are circulating and it is a piece of scientific shorthand to call serum containing, say, antibody to diphtheria bacilli, diphtheria antiserum.
2. It is typical of the comparatively small number of "top-table" immunologists that the team contained, for this work, Eugene Lance, one of the brighter stars on the British scene, who was spending a short time in the United States before starting as a founder-member of the department of immunology at the new National Institute of Clinical Research, Harrow, Middlesex.
3. *Nature*, vol. 227 (August 29, 1970): p. 901.

4 The Early History of the Science

1. *Margin of Safety* (London, 1965), p. 23.
2. *Ibid.*
3. *Ibid.*, p. 25.
4. *Ibid.*, p. 29.

5. Humphrey and White quoting Metchnikoff, *Immunology for Medical Students* (third ed., London, 1969), p. 8.
6. *Op. cit.*, p. 22.

5 The Birth of the Theory of Self

1. Sir Macfarlane Burnet, *Changing Patterns* (London, 1968), pp. 53–54.
2. Burnet, pp. 52–53.
3. *Ibid.*, p. 43.
4. Humphrey and White, pp. 30–31.
5. Humphrey and White, p. 31.
6. The word "clone" is derived from the Greek for a branch or twig.
7. Burnet, p. 213.

6 The Beginning of Modern Immunology

1. *My Life in Science,* BBC Third Programme broadcast, April 23, 1966.
2. (London, 1963), p. vii.
3. *Induction and Intuition in Scientific Thought* (London, 1969), pp. 26 and 32.
4. *Ibid.*, p. 46.
5. Burnet, p. 201.
6. *Ibid.*, p. 245.
7. "Symposium on *Lower Animal Neoplasm* 1969," no. 31 (1969): pp. 41–58.

7 The Development of the Science

1. Robert A. Good, *Journal of Laboratory and Clinical Medicine,* vol. 69 (January 1967): pp. 6–14.
2. Robert A. Good, "Immunologic Reconstitution," *Hospital Practice,* no. 4 (1969): pp. 41–47.

8   *The Importance of Immunology*

1. In the very week of correcting the proofs of this chapter, Professor Clarke and his colleagues published in the *British Medical Journal* (January 11, 1971) the results of their largest test of the new method. It was highly satisfactory and finally proved that the treatment did protect mothers at subsequent pregnancies in large numbers.

9   *The Disadvantages of Immunity*

1. Humphrey and White quoting C. Richet, p. 14.
2. Paul Ehrlich, *Collected Studies on Immunity* (New York, 1906), p. 82.

10   *The Failures of Immunology*

1. *The Common Cold* (London, 1965), p. 31.
2. Quoted from an advance copy of Ian A. McGregor's report, "Immunity to Plasmodial Infection: Consideration of Factors Relevant to Malaria in Man," which the author was allowed to consult.

11   *The Future of Immunology*

1. *"Medicines in the 1990s": A Technological Forecast,* Office of Health Economics no. 162 (London, 1970), p. 9.
2. *Ibid.,* p. 13.
3. From a private interview conducted by the author.
4. There are twenty amino acids and all human protein consists of different numbers of these twenty building blocks arranged in different orders. Three "letters" or "bases" on the nucleic acids give the code for one or another of these amino acids, and this essentially simple system is believed to account for virtually all the structure of living creatures.
5. *Scientific American* (August 1970).
6. *The Immunological Theory of Ageing* (Copenhagen, 1969).

Index

About the Author

David Wilson was born in 1927 in Rugby, Warwick-shire, England. Educated at Ampleforth College, York, and Pembroke College, Cambridge, Mr. Wilson studied mathematics, physics, and history, receiving a B.A. and an M.A. from Cambridge University. A newspaper reporter from 1950 to 1955, he joined the BBC news department in 1956, and has been BBC Science Correspondent since 1963. In addition to broadcasting regularly on BBC radio and television, Mr. Wilson has published a number of articles in *The Listener* and is the author of several books published in Britain. He is married, and the father of four children.

A Note on the Type

The text of this book was set in Caledonia, a Linotype face designed by W. A. Dwiggins. It belongs to the family of printing types called "modern face" by printers—a term used to mark the change in style of type letters that occurred about 1800. Caledonia borders on the general design of Scotch Modern, but is more freely drawn than that letter.

Composed, printed, and bound by
H. Wolff Book Manufacturing Co., Inc.
New York, New York

Typography and binding design
by Virginia Tan